THE WILD
BOY OF
WAUBAMIK

THE WILD BOY OF WAUBAMIK

a memoir

Thom Ernst

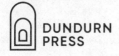

DUNDURN
PRESS

Publisher: Kwame Scott Fraser | Acquiring editor: Russell Smith
Cover designer: Laura Boyle
Cover image: istock.com/IgorBukhlin

Library and Archives Canada Cataloguing in Publication

Title: The wild boy of Waubamik : a memoir / Thom Ernst.
Names: Ernst, Thom, author.
Identifiers: Canadiana (print) 20220271070 | Canadiana (ebook) 2022027116X | ISBN 9781459750876 (softcover) | ISBN 9781459750883 (PDF) | ISBN 9781459750890 (EPUB)
Subjects: LCSH: Ernst, Thom—Childhood and youth. | LCSH: Adult child abuse victims—Ontario—Waubamik—Biography. | LCGFT: Autobiographies.
Classification: LCC HV6626.54.C3 E76 2023 | DDC 362.76092—dc23

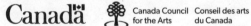

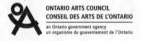 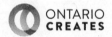

We acknowledge the support of the Canada Council for the Arts and the Ontario Arts Council for our publishing program. We also acknowledge the financial support of the Government of Ontario, through the Ontario Book Publishing Tax Credit and Ontario Creates, and the Government of Canada.

Care has been taken to trace the ownership of copyright material used in this book. The author and the publisher welcome any information enabling them to rectify any references or credits in subsequent editions.

The publisher is not responsible for websites or their content unless they are owned by the publisher.

Printed and bound in Canada.

Dundurn Press
1382 Queen Street East
Toronto, Ontario, Canada M4L 1C9
dundurn.com, @dundurnpress 𝕏 f ⊚

To the Wild Ones

Chapter 1

Dad didn't care much for Catholics, but I wouldn't know how much until my sister married one. Up until then I wasn't even aware we had an opinion on Catholics. Although, looking back, I recall Dad being angry at Bing Crosby for starring as a kindly priest in the 1944 film *Going My Way*.

"There's no such thing as a good Catholic priest," Dad would say.

My sister Anna was marrying James in a Catholic church. On the day of the wedding, Dad announced that he'd be damned if he was going to set foot inside one of those priest-infested monstrosities and that Anna could walk herself down the aisle. Mom told Dad to stop being such a damn fool, get his suit on, and go. That's when Dad stormed out of the house, taking Clancy, his beloved Irish Setter, with him. Uncle Quinnie was in town for the wedding. He called after Dad, but the door had already shut.

Mom said that suited her just fine. She would go to the church on her own. If he decided to show up, he showed up. But she wasn't going to sit around and watch while he ruined their daughter's wedding. Uncle Quinnie told Mom not to worry, that Dad would come around. Mom said she didn't care if he did. But from what I could see from the glimpse I got of Anna in the dining room that had been converted into the bride's dressing room, Anna cared, and so did the bridesmaids who gathered around her. I was just grateful that Mom was angrier with Dad than she was with me for falling and tearing a hole in the knee of my new dress pants.

Later, I was in the kitchen with Uncle Bob, Uncle Quinnie, and Aunt Jean. Valerie, my eldest sister, and her husband, Wayne, were also there. Dad still hadn't come around. The kitchen was small, made smaller with all the aunts and uncles crowded in trying to keep our voices down — except Uncle Bob who, after adding a little extra something in his coffee so he could appropriately celebrate the day, said if something's worth saying aloud, it was worth saying loud. I was the only one seated, having been commanded to *stay put* now that the hole in my pants had been mended. Mom walked in wearing a dress, a necklace, and bright-red lipstick. My uncle commented on how wonderful she looked. Mom offered up an exaggerated grin, meant, I suppose, to be a blushing acceptance. Then she mentioned that Dad's hunting rifle was gone. This new revelation got no more weight than when Wayne had walked in announcing that Dad's car was still in the garage.

Aunt Jean folded her arms. She shook her head and looked to the side where it was impossible for me to read her expression.

Wayne, being the junior of the men in the room, seemed unsure of how much responsibility fell to him in coming up with a solution. But since making decisions is part of Wayne's DNA, he told Valerie, who should have been with the bridesmaids comforting the bride, to go on ahead to the church without him. He suggested, but not with the same authority, that Mom do the same.

"We can't go without him," Valerie said.

"To hell, we can't," said Mom." "Watch me."

But I instead watched my uncles and Wayne take off their dress shoes and put on boots. As far as I knew, Mom was still calling the shots, but the division between male and female, if only by dress code, seemed clear, so I felt obligated to remove my dress shoes, too.

"What do you think you're doing? Leave those on and get in the car." I was surprised by the sharpness in Mom's voice. Perhaps she was still mad at having had to mend my pants. I was disappointed. I would have rather gone with Wayne and my uncles.

"Don't worry, Marg," Uncle Bob said, heading toward the back door. "I'll drag him back by the balls if I have to."

"You can leave him where he is for all I care," Mom yelled back.

In the driveway was a fancy, shiny black car decorated in paper flowers and ribbons. I must have looked quite the gentleman in my suit and tie and mended dress pants, for the man who stood beside the car opened the back door. It would have been rude had I not climbed in, but just as the smell of a clean and leathery interior took hold of me, I felt a tug at the back of my pants.

"Haul your butt out of there. We're taking the Rambler." Mom again. The man holding the door laughed and said something about me looking so sharp he thought I was the groom. I wondered how many other people I would be able to fool into thinking I was the groom. "Get in the car, in the back." Mom pointed to the Rambler. "Aunt Jean is riding with us."

I sulked with enough intensity to leave no misunderstanding as to how unfair it was that I should not be allowed to go with Uncle Bob and look for the rifle.

I was told several times during the ride to sit down. It was an unusual request, given the number of road trips I spent standing with my head leaning between the driver and the front seat passenger. That way, I wouldn't be left out of the conversation, *plus* I got a better view because I was that much closer to the front windshield.

I asked Mom if she had any gum in her purse, or perhaps a peppermint Life Saver. She said that if she had to tell me to sit properly in the back seat one more time, she'd stop the car and tie me in. I sat back, firing angry vibes into the rear-view mirror. Aunt Jean rooted through her purse and found a roll of fruit-flavour Life Savers and handed me the entire roll. She said I could keep them. The first one was red, the best flavour. I popped the red Life Saver into my mouth and watched as the landscape changed from farm-land to suburb.

There wasn't a lot of chatting between Mom and Aunt Jean, and then I heard Mom say that she hoped Dad didn't do anything stupid, to which Aunt Jean replied, "It's a bit late for that."

We arrived at the church where a young man, whom I recognized as one of James's brothers, greeted us at the door, took Mom's arm, and walked us to the front of the church. People stared as if they knew we didn't belong in such an extravagant place and were whispering their disapproval as we passed. Indeed, I had never seen a place as extravagant as a Catholic church with its stained-glass windows, ornate lights hanging from high ceilings, painted statues of Jesus and his mother, altars covered in red-and-white satin, and a cross as big as a house. If this wasn't where God lived, then it's where he summered.

A man stood at the front of the church wearing white robes and a sash over his shoulders. I asked Mom if that was the minister, and she told me that he's called a *priest* — a word that left her mouth with some disdain. Although he didn't look friendly, I thought he looked important, and I couldn't understand a word he said, even when he wasn't speaking Catholic. A boy, also in a white robe, stood with him. I figured the boy must be the priest's son. The boy held up a bowl in which the priest dipped his fingers then took them out, shaking off the excess water. The boy handed the priest a towel, the priest dried his hand and gave the towel back. I was annoyed that the priest's son got to be part of my sister's wedding and I didn't.

James — the groom — also stood at the front. He stood soldier-straight, rubbing one hand against his pant leg as if hopelessly trying to remove something damp and sticky off his palms. He looked sharp in a dark tuxedo, smiling awkwardly at whoever he made eye contact with.

Uncle Bob walked up to Mom and said something into her ear. Mom's expression didn't change. She whispered something back to Uncle Bob, which I didn't hear. Uncle Bob nodded, placed his hand on Mom's back, and left.

Soon after, the music started — a gentle, familiar melody that I couldn't name. The congregation rose, which made it impossible for me to see anything past a forest of butts and beltlines. Mom whispered that a procession was coming down the aisle and Valerie was in the lead. A procession, I imagined, was something like a parade but with people you recognized. I saw Valerie once the procession reached the front of the church. Valerie walked arm-in-arm with her husband, Wayne. They moved slowly as though the next step they took was more important than the one that just passed. A sombre march, in contrast with their happy and nervous faces. Next came Anna's friend Claudette with Don, James's older brother. They, too, moved with precise, synchronized steps. The last in this procession of paired-off couples was my cousin Sue, who shared her arm with James's youngest brother, the other Wayne.

The couples unlocked arms as they reached the front of the church, the women to the left and the men to the right. The music stopped. Someone in the congregation coughed. The priest looked down at James, then to the back of the church, and nodded. The music began again, filling the church with the elongated notes of the wedding march pumped from a pipe organ, as if announcing the arrival of God.

People shifted to get a better look. A rumble of approving voices rolled like a summer storm behind the flash of cameras. Carol Chapman — the little girl who lived next door and my occasional playmate — four years old, diminutive, dressed in white with a tiara-like veil attached to her hair, moved down the aisle grasping a bouquet of flowers, keeping her head facing forward as she had been firmly instructed to do, while her eyes darted from side to side, catching glimpses of the smiles and camera lightning flashes along the way.

And then came the bride, my sister Anna, in a princess gown. A veil draped over her head, but one that left her teenage beauty, a face, stoic and uncertain, in full view.

On her arm was Dad, wearing the suit Mom laid out for him and the boutonniere reserved for the father of the bride.

Uncle Bob, Uncle Quinnie, and Wayne had found him standing with Clancy behind Montag's barn. He said he was hunting rabbits. But the rabbits stayed hidden, and Dad hadn't done anything stupid. I wondered if Uncle Bob had to drag him by the balls.

Dad did not smile. His eyes darted, not to catch the glimpses of friends and family, but to avoid them. He stopped at the front and handed Anna over to James like he was passing a cheque. Then he joined Mom and me in the front pew. Mom motioned for me to slide down and make room for Dad. Neither Mom nor Dad spoke.

The priest moved his hands over the congregation and mumbled a few incoherent Catholic words. He told the congregation to kneel, and they did, even the Protestants. I wanted to kneel, too, because how often do you get to kneel in church wearing your best suit, but my kneeling made Dad so angry that I thought he would reach over Mom and clout me a good one or, worse, yell at me right there in front of all these Catholics, so Mom hefted me up by the arm and shoved my butt back onto the pew. She sure didn't need me getting

Dad all riled up in front of everyone. Or maybe they were afraid I'd put another hole in the knee of my pants. The ceremony ended and with it the struggle to not be Catholic in a Catholic Church.

After, there was a party at the Blue Moon Tavern in Petersburg. Dad's mood changed for the better — Uncle Bob said that he just needed to get a few drinks in him. The Catholics, except for James and his family, kept to themselves. I didn't know who was a Catholic and who wasn't, so when the music started, I danced with everyone. I discovered I had a natural groove, and all the attention I lost for not being part of the ceremony I got back from an unconscious display of my wicked dance moves.

The night ended with a strange and ominous occurrence: a meteorite streaked across the sky, then vanished in a burst of light that briefly turned night into day. A spectacle that stopped the party. The gasps and awes from the partiers rose above the sound of Tom Jones singing "Save the Last Dance for Me." I had no idea what it was that I had just seen. Wayne said it was a meteorite. Mom said it was a falling star, and I should have made a wish when I saw it, but it's too late now. And Uncle Bob told me it was a flying saucer and that by morning we'd be overrun by martians.

Whatever it was, meteorite, falling star, or flying saucer, all I know is that it came from outer space.

I went to bed thinking that the world was about to end. It didn't, at least not in any way I expected. But with Anna gone my world was about to get darker in ways too subtle to notice, too insidious to recognize.

Chapter 2

- - - - - - - - - -

With Anna living with James, Dad seemed motivated to spend more time with me. Prior to this our relationship, though not exactly strained, had been distant. Now there were rides in the belly of the wheelbarrow with me holding on to its metal edges as Dad raced over the tiny moguls in the lawn that ran from the garden to the garage. There was more time for him to stop whatever he was doing, working in the garden or raking the leaves, to push me on the swing high enough to worry that I'd be flung up and over the bars. There were the helicopter rides where I was held by my arms or legs, sometimes an arm and a leg, and spun around until airborne. He would land me safely back to earth, uninjured, always careful not to hurt me. And there were piggyback rides where I was jostled and bounced down the hall and back again. Even better were shoulder rides where I suddenly was taller than anyone in the room.

There were games of crazy eights on days Dad worked the night shift at Uniroyal. I would rush home from school to get as many hands in as possible before Dad left for the factory. It hardly mattered that I'd lose almost every game or that losing would set me up for some hard-core ribbing. Just part of the game.

"You're never going to beat me," Dad would say, staking claim to the victor's right to ridicule. But he was wrong, as I eventually became something of a crazy eights champion. And the good-natured ribbing I learned so well by his example became mine to dispense. Only my skills at bantering weren't refined enough to not cause offence. My friendly jabs didn't come across as being all that friendly, leaving Dad growing red-faced and sputtering his frustrations through tight thin lips. I couldn't be sure that his burst of anger wasn't also part of this sportsmanlike rigmarole of playful insults and harmless threats until he hurled the cards across the room and demanded I go upstairs and get out of his sight.

I protested to Mom, arguing that winning a card game is hardly a punishable offence. But Mom took Dad's side.

"No one likes to lose all the time," she said. "It would be nice if you were to let him win once in a while."

There didn't seem to be much logic in playing to lose, and since that would be our last game of crazy eights together, I never got the chance to test Mom's theory.

But there is one memory that I choose to keep close, a moment I've decided to believe is an example of Dad sincerely acting as a parent. I was sleeping on the living room couch because the couch is where I stayed when sick, probably because of the proximity of the washroom. I woke feeling nauseous, so I cried out for Mom, but it was Dad who came. He sat at the foot of the couch and took my hand. I remember the warmth of his hand as healing, calming. I fell back to sleep but woke up again to see that my dad was still there, still holding my hand, his eyes closed. Sleeping. I looked at him. The nausea had passed. I closed my eyes and slept comfortably for the rest of the night.

But despite the good things, there remained a disconnect — an emotional distance that I was unable to cross. It was around then, with some help from Mom, that I began to understand my failings as a son, and that perhaps Dad's moodiness and distance from me was not his fault alone.

Mom was always frank with her explanations.

"Your Dad wanted a son — someone he could play sports with and who'd help him around the house. So, we got you." Mom was stirring a large pot of whole tomatoes directly from our garden in preparation of a spaghetti sauce that would simmer through the night and into the next day. Mom's spaghetti sauce was an event meal, given that her cooking ranged mostly from Depression-era bland to Depression-era not-quite-as bland. Recalling this even now is to bring back the aroma of fresh garden-grown tomatoes blending in with herbs and spices and left to simmer on the stovetop. "But you're not interested in hockey, or any sport from what we can tell. The only things that interest you are the movies."

Well, movies, yes. But I would add reading and writing — anything involving a story. Mom had me pegged, and so I committed to being the kid Dad wanted. My starting point was the sports pages of the *Kitchener-Waterloo Record* and watching televised events, mostly hockey, hoping for a sports breakthrough that would open my eyes to the thrill of competition. I picked a favourite team: the Boston Bruins was as good as any. And I picked a favourite player, Bobby Orr. Bobby Orr was a Bruin, and, like me, he was born in Parry Sound. But despite all efforts, a true love for sports never happened and I eventually had to give up hockey and go back to the movies.

What I hadn't expected was for Dad to show interest in what interested me. He bought me books, read my writing — even the poems — and best of all, there were trips to the drive-in movies. We watched a Clint Eastwood Man with No Name movie marathon:

A Fistful of Dollars; For a Few Dollars More; The Good, the Bad and the Ugly. I loved every one of them, but Dad thought they were too violent. He didn't like violence in the movies. "There's enough real violence in the world without putting fake violence in the movies," he would say.

Dad preferred the Carry On gang movies. Mom would come along for those. Even Mom had to laugh at the scenes where the buxom blond gets caught naked and frantically tries to cover up. Nudity was fine so long as it was British.

Things continued to go well but for a few minor bumps along the way, things of which I'd been convinced were overreactions on my part. Like the time Dad nearly drowned me with an economy-sized bottle of Pepsi.

We were at the Fairview Drive-In. The movie was *Dear Heart*, starring Glenn Ford. We brought a bottle of Pepsi with us because, according to Mom, what they charged at the concession booth amounted to nothing less than highway robbery. I had a cup, but Dad was not about to leave me with a cup full of Pepsi in the back seat of his car. And so, he twisted the metal cap allowing a *phssst* sound to escape the bottle, turned from his place in the driver's seat, and told me to move forward so that I was in the middle of the back seat between my parents. I reached for the bottle, but Dad pulled it back. I couldn't be trusted to not spill it.

"I think he can manage holding a bottle of Pepsi," said Mom, eyes still on the screen.

"Better not," said Dad. "I don't want Pepsi spilled all over the place." So, Dad held the bottle to my lips and tipped it so that the brown carbonated syrup flowed into my mouth and down my throat. It was a nice gesture, to offer a refreshing summer drink to your son. And since neither Pepsi nor Coca-Cola were common household items, this was indeed something special. One more thing for me to be grateful for.

I raised my hand to let Dad know I'd had enough, moved my fingers to the glass neck of the bottle, trying to push the bottle away, but Dad held the bottle in place. He continued pouring, watching, smiling. I had no choice but to keep chugging, not wanting to spill Pepsi on my pyjamas or, worse, on the back seat upholstery. I'd had enough but that message wasn't getting to Dad. He kept smiling and pouring. The bubbles burned my throat and pricked the inside of my cheeks. I did my best to indicate that I was done, that I couldn't drink anymore, that it was beginning to hurt, that Pepsi fizz was building up in my stomach and the back of my throat. Dad found this all very funny. And to be fair, I must have been quite the sight what with my eyes bugging out, panicking while Dad kept laughing, tilting the bottle higher.

Mom looked at me and then at Dad.

"Clare," she said, "he's telling you he's had enough." But Dad wasn't ready for the fun to end. The timing was important or else there would be quite the mess in the car and the fault wouldn't be mine. Unless it was.

"Clare, you're drowning the kid." Mom's laugh seemed nervous, not, I don't think, because of my discomfort but because this family outing was going well, and Mom was not about to change the tone of the evening by scolding Dad too harshly.

Dad's smile had an unconfirmed menace to it, the kind that if you were to point it out to someone, they could just as easily not see it as to see it. It could be the bright and friendly, cheerful smile of a family man having a wonderful time with his family, or the sinister grin of someone withholding a nasty secret. Mom scolded him gently like he was a mischievous jokester, a clown, a lovable prankster who was, perhaps, taking the joke a breath too far.

"Clare, he's going throw up all over the back seat of the car."

And then Dad stopped. He would have had to eventually, so he chose then. I gasped and coughed and wheezed, trying to regain whatever oxygen had been lost. Mom told me to open the door and lean outside if I thought I was going to be sick.

In the end it was made clear that had I been sick, or spewed Pepsi in the car, it would have been my fault when all I had to do was put my tongue up against the opening in the bottleneck and simply stop swallowing. It was obvious when I thought on it, but when it was happening, when my stomach was swelling up like the gullet of an over-filled wineskin and I was sputtering carbonated foam from the corners of my mouth like water from a compressed garden hose — the obvious wasn't so obvious. In time, instinct would have taken over and I would have moved my mouth, gasping and vomiting Pepsi all over the backseat while the rest of the bottle emptied on top of me. That wouldn't have gone over too well, but at least I was in no real threat of drowning.

And at least it gave Mom and Dad a good laugh.

"Did you see the look on his face?" Dad said. "I thought his eyes were going to pop right out of his head."

"Honestly, and all he had to do was put his tongue up against the bottle and stop the flow. Doesn't even know enough to stop drinking when he's full."

Mom and Dad. What jokesters.

A few weeks later Mom unexpectedly took ill, and for the first time I would be left in the sole care of my dad. It would be then, without Mom to intervene or distract, that the demons my dad had been keeping in check were allowed to run free.

Chapter 3

-- -- -- -- -- -- --

I was invisible on the morning Mom left. I simply woke and could not be seen. Had I disappeared, and the police came to the house and asked, "When was the last time anyone saw Thom," not a soul would be able to say. Even Dad, whose procedural efforts to prepare breakfast made him seem more robot than human, would not have been able to remember when he saw me last.

"Where's Mom?" I asked, not caring for this unstructured switch of parental duties, although the steaming cup of Nescafé instant coffee sitting next to my bowl of cornflakes was a curious but not unpleasant addition.

"In bed. Leave her be." But Mom didn't sleep in. Dad had yet to look at me or say anything that didn't sound like a command. Clancy pushed against Dad's legs, looking for a pat or recognition. "What do you want?" he said to the dog. "You've been fed, go lie down."

Clancy did as she was told, looking up at her master, hurt and dejected. When I left the breakfast table, I stopped to pat Clancy and remind her that she's a good girl. Clancy's tail thumped approval, but I was a poor second to Dad. I went upstairs quietly so as not to disturb Mom. Her door was opened enough I could see her lying on her back, her eyes closed, one arm folded over the top of her head. She was not sleeping.

When I left the house for school, I said goodbye without anyone saying goodbye back. I'd like to say that on that day I was a distracted student, unable to focus because all my thoughts were on my sick mother, who before now had never so much as complained of a headache. But I don't know if that's true. I cannot recall if I thought much about Mom at all that day. When I came home, Valerie's car was in the driveway. Dad's car, too. He had not gone to work.

Valerie was at the kitchen sink, soaking a washcloth. I waited before I said anything; this only seemed fitting given the room's mood. Valerie was not here for a visit; that much was clear. She was not the friendly, welcoming Valerie I was familiar with. Valerie noticed me, but my presence was observed as if by accident.

"Thom, go on upstairs and find something to do," Valerie told me. I was being dismissed.

"What about dinner?" The question came out as naturally as if the responsibility of dinner had always been Valerie's.

"I'll get dinner started in a bit. Mom's not feeling well," she said and carried the wet cloth into the front room.

I passed through the kitchen into the hallway, where I saw Mom lying on the couch in the front room. Her eyes were closed, but she was not sleeping. Dad sat beside her holding her hand as he had held mine only a year before. At some point, Mom had got dressed, yet remained as I left her in that morning, with an arm bent over her forehead, shielding the light from her eyes.

"What's wrong?" I asked, but Dad sent me to my room. I was startled by the confusion and fear in his voice, and yet I couldn't obey. Not immediately. Instead, I watched as Valerie entered the room and placed the wet cloth on Mom's head. Mom moved her hand to hold the fabric in place, managing a weak "thank you."

"Is she okay?"

Dad didn't answer.

"Go on upstairs, Thom," Valerie said. "I'll come for you soon."

"Is that Thom?" Mom asked as though talking from a dream. No answer for her either. Not even from me.

I headed toward the stairwell when I heard Mom say, with urgency, that she needed to be taken to the washroom. *Mom is asking for help. Mom never asks for help. Mom never gets ill.*

I stood at the bottom of the stairs across from the washroom. Mom came down the hall, Valerie on one side, Dad on the other, supporting her as they guided her toward the bathroom like a blindfolded, kidnapped victim being shuffled from one hiding place to another. Mom kept her head down. One hand reached past Valerie, brushing along the hallway wall, supporting slow, deliberate steps.

The bathroom door closed behind them. Mom moaned.

"It's okay, Mom," I heard Valerie say.

Moments later, Mom's overnight bag was packed, and I, no doubt pumped with inappropriate and unveiled excitement, was sent to spend the night at my friend Doug's house.

* * *

I don't know why Mrs. Chapman thought it necessary to bring a casserole. Casseroles were for funerals. Mom was sick, but not casserole sick. Then again, I couldn't really say how sick Mom was or why she was rushed to the hospital. I was told that Mom is in the hospital for reasons that don't concern me and that she was in good hands and will be home when she gets home (so I might as well stop asking). That was all the explanation an eight-year-old needs for why he will be motherless for the next several weeks.

I stood back from the door and listened to Dad's stammering attempts to tell Mrs. Chapman that Mom won't be gone for more than a few more days, and thanks for the casserole, but we're good. Mrs. Chapman wouldn't hear of it. She insisted Dad take the casserole; it was already made. Besides, even if Mom wasn't dying, she's in the hospital. Apparently, casseroles were just as good for hospital stays as funerals. Mrs. Chapman shoved the casserole dish into Dad's midriff as if she were handing off a football. Dad had little choice but to grab the dish or let it crash against the concrete step. Mrs. Chapman won the battle of the casseroles, and Dad, not having the skills to accept generosity with good grace, offered a clumsy and unconvincing thank you.

The casserole filled the kitchen with a comfortable smell of stability, a promising reprieve from Dad's culinary repertoire of fried eggs, cheese sandwiches, Heinz pork 'n beans, canned soup, and liver and onions. But it was not to be. Dad didn't care for fancy foods like casseroles. We weren't fancy people, and we didn't eat things cooked in other peoples' kitchens; for all we know it could be loaded with crazy fixings like paprika or parmesan cheese. Or possibly Dad was embarrassed that Mrs. Chapman went to the trouble of making a casserole without the decency of anyone dying.

He crammed the dish, still warm and steaming, into the freezer. It stayed there until weeks later when it was rediscovered as a mystery dish covered in freezer burns.

The aroma of the casserole was soon masked by the distinct smell of liver and onions burning in the frying pan. Dad had his back to me, attending to the sliced onions, not sautéed but fried, pushing them about the pan, making sure they were evenly burned on all sides. What would have happened if Mrs. Chapman's instincts were right? What if Mom's illness did warrant a casserole? What then? Would I be forever subjected to eating undercooked slabs of meat and cremated vegetables?

"Your mother's fine," Dad grumbled, his frustration not with me but with this new task of having to cook. "Stop asking. It's a woman's thing. That's all you need to know."

A woman's thing? One more confounding addition to a growing list of questions.

It didn't take long for the strict regime Mom so stringently enforced of an early bedtime, no snacks before dinner, no sugar before bed, plus limited access to what could be watched on television, began to fall apart. I was clearly taking advantage of Dad's inability to maintain structure, but if Dad wasn't going to enforce the rules, I wasn't going to remind him. But it's not that Dad simply forgot or neglected the rules, he actively put the rules aside, encouraging me to grab the chips from the cupboard or the ice cream from the fridge, letting me watch *Rowan & Martin's Laugh-In*, *The Dean Martin Show*, and even *The Tonight Show Starring Johnny Carson*.

One night we were in the living room. For reasons that I can no longer remember and would likely not make sense to me even if I did, neither of us thought to turn on the television. With the television off, the living room became a sombre, cavernous chamber lit by the single glow from a standing lamp behind Mom's easy chair.

That night, Dad sat in Mom's chair — uneasy in the easy chair — his entire body an unnatural fit in the indentation left by Mom. His shape sank into the oversized cushion, his whole body sulking. As unaccustomed as Dad was to charity, he was less accustomed to comfort. His arms rested stiffly on the cushioned armrests, fingers curled over the rounded edges. He had the appearance of an unfit leader defiantly clinging to a throne he feared would be taken from him.

I was talking, filling the bleak void with the chatter of my play, giving voice to imaginary drivers of the die-cast sports cars going top speed down a plastic stretch of flexible orange highway and squealing their tires crossing a carpet terrain. Dad said nothing — a man lost in the thoughts that brewed and twisted inside him. Dad's face was hidden in the shadows, his head drooped on his shoulders. He watched me, the proverbial hawk, leaving me as ... what? The field mouse?

I was glad to have my Hot Wheels. I'd rather be playing with my G.I. Joes, but Dad disapproved of boys playing with dolls, even if those dolls are equipped with combat gear and hand grenades and had a Kung Fu grip.

I suspected his dislike of G.I. Joes had something to do with the story about him and Uncle Quinnie being chased from the boys' section of the schoolyard to the girls' section because Oma refused to cut their hair or dress them in anything but short pants, no matter how much their father pleaded on his sons' behalf. So, despite my own protests, my hair was kept to a bristly, unstylish brush cut, and flamboyant fashions like bell-bottoms and billowy-sleeved pirate shirts were outlawed. And I was not, under any circumstances, allowed to play with dolls, even if I called them action figures. Dad was just looking out for my masculinity.

I was lost in a world of reckless-driving hot rodders when Dad spoke. Though soft and uncommonly serene, the suddenness of his voice jolted me out of my play and back into the living room. His question caught me off guard. "What kind of car is that?" he asked.

What kind of what is what? His words had meaning, but I lost all ability to decipher them. Then, as if capable of registering my confusion, the cold metallic object in my hand responded on my behalf.

Me, said the object in my hand. *He wants to know about me. I'm a Redline Custom Volkswagen with a front exposed engine. Tell him.*

I held the car up. "It's a Redline Custom Volkswagen with a front exposed engine."

"A what?" he asked. "Bring it here."

I walked to the chair, the Volkswagen in hand. Dad took the car from me and turned it in his hand, looking at the undercast engine. He spun the wheels.

"Wow. This sure is a nice car. Where did you get this one?" The question felt forced, drummed up out of a need to hold my attention. It didn't seem like questions that needed or even wanted answers. Not even then. But I answered, anyway.

"Al," I told him, arbitrarily naming the man who had been dating, and who would later marry, my cousin Patty.

"Al!" he said, as if this was a shocking yet incredible revelation. "When did Al get this for you?"

"I don't know. One time."

Dad looked to the Hot Wheels collection on the carpet area where I played.

"Show me another of your favourites."

Another favourite? Even the Volkswagen with the exposed engine was randomly selected, but he wanted another favourite? I scanned the floor for a car sporty enough to warrant being called a favourite. I chose the Batmobile, which flickered with a retractable plastic flame pushing in and out of the exhaust whenever the vehicle was in motion. I brought the toy to him.

"What does it do?" He took the car and held it at eye level.

"It shoots flames out the back."

"No? It can't do that, can it?" One of Dad's great talents was to feign dismay.

"It can," I said, pleased to have the chance to amaze him.

"No, I don't believe it. Show me," Dad said, slapping his lap, showing me plenty of room for a young chap like me. It was strange; maybe it shouldn't have been, but it was. I couldn't recall having ever sat on his lap.

"Come on up," he repeated, handing me back the car. "Show me how it works."

There remained the problem of manoeuvring myself onto his lap, so Dad helped. He leaned over and hefted me up, but I was too large to lift off the ground. He dragged me onto his lap.

"Wow, you got heavy," he said.

Did I? But the thought, which wasn't a thought but a voice, was not mine. I turned to see who else was in the room.

A boy. Younger than me. He was standing by the entrance to the hallway. In his hand looked to be a doll without a head. It was not a G.I. Joe. The boy's hair was matted and unwashed. There were holes in the knees of his pants, his knees scratched and bruised. Dad didn't see him. Neither did Clancy, who lay nearby, watching and thinking whatever thoughts a dog thinks.

The thought-voice continued. It was a small but precise voice. And yet it made sense that I was the only one who heard. And the only one who saw.

Yeah, well, kids tend to do that. They get heavy, especially ones who've been stuffed with candy and ice cream and soft drinks and are sleep deprived. Maybe that's how he liked them — heavy, complacent, and lethargic with no fight in them. Or perhaps you're too fucking old to be sitting on your Dad's lap. I don't get it. Why now? You weren't sitting on his lap at four or five or six, so why suddenly at eight?

Dad held me in place with one hand resting on my hip. I tried to ignore the boy. It was nice having my dad's attention — but on his lap? I thought the time for lap-sitting had come and gone. It was awkward, but I embraced the moment, fearing that doing otherwise would alienate him forever. I was distracted from my discomfort by focusing on the Batmobile. I spun the back wheels. Tiny plastic flames bobbed in and out of the exhaust pipes.

"Wow. That's something," Dad said. "Let me try."

I handed him the car, and, as with the Volkswagen, he studied the cast-iron chassis top and bottom. Then, a test drive for quality, he ran the vehicle up and down my leg. Did he like the Batmobile or not? He didn't say. He put the Batmobile down, balanced on an unused armrest. His eyes closed. I thought he might have fallen asleep. Was I supposed to get down now? But his arm kept me in place, so I wouldn't — or couldn't — slip off.

Then Dad asked if I was ticklish.

Ticklish?

"I don't know," I said. It had been a while since Dad had me pinned while roughhousing on the living room carpet. I would struggle, fiercely but playfully, to free myself from his grip.

And then, helpless, he'd have me squealing for mercy while he poked around my ribs, armpits, and neck, and the most torturous of all, immobilized me while he attacked the bottom of my feet. But that was long ago.

"Let's find out," he said, going for my ribs. I laughed because tickling is meant to be fun, and no one wants to be a spoilsport. The tickle was sharp and set my nerves and muscles into a painful spasm. I struggled to get free because that's part of the game, but his grip got tighter. Then he asked if I knew where boys are most ticklish?

I did. The bottom of the feet.

No, that was not the answer.

"Yeah," he conceded. "Feet are ticklish. But I know a place that's more ticklish than that."

"Armpits."

"No," he said. "Want me to show you?"

Say no, said the boy in the hallway.

Dad showed me, and when he did, I reacted when his fingers reached down my lap, danced along the inside of my thigh, inching upwards until he reached the most ticklish part ever so lightly. I leaped from his lap, managed to break from his grip, and landed on the floor. Dad laughed the way someone might laugh to console a frightened child, assuring them that there was no reason for such an overreaction. He was just showing me, that was all.

I laughed, too, as if being told a dirty joke, but a joke no eight-year-old wanted to hear from their father. Dad invited me back up on his lap.

"It won't happen again," he said. But why were his eyes closed?

Go to your room. Shut the door. Prop a chair against the door. Go to Mrs. Chapman's — take the casserole. Go to Doug's — watch horror movies. Go. Do something.

I crawled onto Dad's lap. After all, he said it won't happen again. But it did, and again, I jumped from his lap. Again, I laughed though it was less funny than before. Dad laughed, too, because isn't this a silly game? A little silly tickle game, getting such a big reaction. So funny. So ticklish. He called me back. I said no, but it was not a refusal, and he knew it. Because, of course, whatever it felt like, wasn't what was happening. It couldn't be.

"Oh," he said, demolishing my resistance with an elongated vowel, "I'm not going to do it again."

"Promise?"

"Scout's honour." He held up three fingers solidifying the oath.

I crawled on his lap because no one breaks a scout's honour. He kept his promise. For a while, but not a long while. Then he gripped me so I was unable to budge. He wanted to show me just how ticklish it can get. This next time, it didn't tickle, but I had to laugh or risk being on his lap forever. Dad said not to worry. He said all boys did this. He said it was relaxing, that it felt good. But I didn't feel good. But not to worry, he was teaching me how it was done. How to relax. That was what fathers did.

Then Dad got tired of the tickle game. He had a new idea.

"Hey," he said. "You like to read books, don't you?"

Chapter 4

- - - - - - - - - - -

The book was a paperback titled *Northwest Passion*. It was hidden in the bottom drawer of Dad's desk, shoved beneath a seven-year span of returned income tax forms. On the book's jacket was a vividly charged image of several beefy men drawn to look like lumberjacks or French voyageurs leering over several buxom women who are laughing drunkenly at the men's attempts to strong-arm them into something they are up for in the first place. Dad told me that the men and women on the cover of *Northwest Passion* were having fun, but I thought their faces seemed crazed and vicious and starved. Dad read to me his favourite parts, including a chapter where two women kiss and touch each other in the front seat of a car. The details of what they do, the older woman coaxing, the younger woman reluctant but soon swooning in ecstasy, made my body shiver. I was drowning in a new kind of sin and didn't even try to stay afloat.

And then in the moment of a touch, a slight twitch of his fingers, my world changed forever. I now knew too much to ever hope I could return to normal. I drifted toward my room as if it might be the one place that still made sense. But sense knew better than to stick around. The hour was well beyond reason. I had been dropped in a pocket of time that should not exist, suspended between too late and too early. I was numb to whatever adrenalin carried me forward. In my belly was a lightness I only now equate with the sensation of no longer being part of this Earth, and if there ever was such a thing as a soul, then I was sure that mine had got up and left.

There was only the light from a desk lamp bleeding through the crack of the open door of my parent's room. My feet were bare, of that I'm sure, but I couldn't tell you now if the floor beneath me was wood or carpet. The details of that night unfurled like smoke, twisting and turning in on itself, a snake swallowing its tail.

I climbed onto my bed, imagining myself to be a wounded cat looking for a proper place to die. I took to my mattress like a cast-away to a life raft, wanting more from it than it could possibly give: warmth, comfort, and a magical ability to roll back time. My body was fouled, rotting, and stained. My skin was ablaze in shame and confusion, though I wouldn't have known its cause then. And I remember that I thought of nothing, because once you've been shoved off the edge of the Earth, nothing is the best you can hope for, except maybe for hitting the bottom of an endless drop. I died in that fall but rose again to become one of the living dead.

And then I saw the Wild Boy.

The Wild Boy watched me from an unlit corner of my room, but his face stood out from the shadows. The same shadowed look I had seen when he stood in the hallway downstairs. He sat in my grandfather's chair, the chair that didn't mesh with the rest of the furniture in the house, and so was relegated to my room to clash with the other mismatched, abandoned pieces cluttering my space. The sudden appearance of a scrawny little boy in my dead grandpa's chair should have made me jump, but it didn't. Too much had already happened. It may have been like how Mom felt when, at twelve, she saw an angel outside her bedroom window. It came down, she said, to quiet a howling dog mourning at the foot of a street lamp over the loss of its owner. Mom's angel never touched the ground. Instead, it hovered by the street lamp, reached out with what looked like a staff and gently touched the dog. According to Mom, the dog stopped howling, tucked its tail between its legs, and left. Then Mom watched as the angel returned to the sky. Mom told me she didn't feel fear, only an indescribable peace. I didn't fear the boy, but neither did I feel an indescribable peace. A chill ran through me, not from seeing him in my room, but a chill from knowing that he could see me.

"I know you," I told him.

The Wild Boy smiled. He nodded his head, in a gesture seemingly beyond his years, appreciative of the recognition, like a celebrity who doesn't expect to go unnoticed.

I did know him. In the hallway, I might have recognized him sooner had he not appeared so suddenly. Before then, the Wild Boy existed only in the stories told, usually at my pleading, from people who had less to do with him than I did.

I waited for the Wild Boy to talk. I didn't have to wait long.

I don't like the way you smile, he said. *It's weird.* His voice was disarmingly young, the undeveloped tone of a child but with full adult use of cadence and skillful intonations.

My smile. I hadn't realized that I'd been grinning. Once I'd been made aware of it, the grin grew wider until the corners of my mouth ached. I turned my head as I would if I wanted to avoid any outside triggers influencing an inappropriate response, like a friend trying to make you laugh in church.

It's the smile of a bullshitter. I think, maybe, of a coward who's cried uncle one too many times. But that's not the worst thing about your smile. Do you want to know the worst thing about your smile?

I didn't.

The worst thing is that you look willing to take it. That you're condemned to live life rolling with the punches. A whole life of grinning and bearing it. Look at me, he says. Look at me.

I looked. The Wild Boy was no longer in the chair but sitting atop my dresser like a nursery-rhyme character on the edge of a wall. It was in keeping with the myriad of strange things that day. *Don't you want to tell the world how pissed off you are?*

The world. Did the world need to know?

Don't you want to tell the world to go fuck itself?

I cringed. I didn't need to say anything. The Wild Boy seemed to know me better than I did. I wanted to tell him that if I'm too young to hear the f-word, he's too young to say it.

Whoa, he said, his tiny voice taking stock of my reaction, *I surprise you. Is it that I said "fuck"? Not a word you use, is it?*

In the next room, the desk lamp turned off.

The Wild Boy looked as if calculating his following words. *I think you should use it. I think now is a perfect time. You'd be surprised how much it helps.* But I already knew, and the Wild Boy knew, too, that I couldn't let the world find out. That the anger had to stay here. And then the boy leaped from the dresser. He walked over to the bed, crawled beside me, and got under the covers. He leaned into my ear and, in the sweet, gentle lilt of an infant cooing, let loose with a litany of the foulest curse words I had ever heard.

It was comforting.

I woke with the dream-swearing still ricocheting in my head. But it was not words seeping from my dream into reality, but rather words from reality seeping into my dream. The Chapman brothers, Scott and Paul, were outside cussing each other over whose turn it was to feed the chickens. It felt absurd that something as familiar as brothers bickering over their chores was still possible in the world I woke up in. And yet I was comforted, somewhat, that life goes on. *The more things change, the more they stay the same,* Mom would say.

It took an effort to lift my head from the pillow to see if the Wild Boy was still here. He was gone, as I suppose I knew he would be. The clothes I had thrown on the chair were now on the floor. I dropped my head back onto the pillow. There was nothing left in me to move: I was tired, lazy, and scared. I thought that if I were to stay in bed, if I concocted a way to never have to move again, I could pretend nothing had happened. I could lie there forever smiling. And people would approach my parents and ask, "What the hell is wrong with your kid?"

"Not a clue," my parents would tell them. "He just woke up one morning grinning like a damn fool, and he's been grinning ever since."

"Damn fool kid."

"Well, he's adopted." And that would be all the explanation anyone needed.

Chapter 5

- - - - - - - - - - -

I was four when I was first told about my adoption. I took the news surprisingly well. Mostly, because when Mom sat me in the kitchen, handed me a carton of animal cookies, and told me that *I was adopted*, I thought she said that *I was a doctor*. I knew enough about doctors to know they could be imposing and impressive creatures of authority, and I was okay with that. But as I worked through the box of animal cookies, biting off the heads of giraffes and lions, with Mom telling me how lucky I was and that there were hundreds of boys and girls without mommies and daddies who'd give their right arm to be in my shoes (Mom would have had quite the impressive collection of body parts for all the limbs people would have given to be as lucky as me), I became less enamoured with the idea. I imagined an image stolen directly from the pages of my Children's Bible where generic rosy-cheeked children, who for no discernible reason faced west with their heads tilted toward the sky, stood aimlessly beneath a ray of light as if world was not enough for them. Motherless children: lost but pure and entirely holy.

"Where are their mommies?" I asked. I could tell my question pleased Mom, if only because it indicated that some of what she was saying was beginning to sink in.

"Well," she replied, "some of their mothers died."

The notion of a dead mother horrified me.

"Did my mommy die?" I asked.

"No, your mother was too young to care for you properly, and God knows where your father took off to."

There it was, the resentment resonating in my mother's voice toward lost fathers; the fathers who chose to be lost, which I understood to include my own. Villains unworthy of concern or curiosity.

She continued, "Your mother couldn't care for you, so we took you." Granted, there may have been a slight variation on her words, like "so we will care for you," or "so she gave you to us," but the overall take-away was a feeling of being shuffled from one home to another. It's unclear, but it was likely at that point I realized that being adopted had nothing to do with being a doctor. Soon after, and without warning, I threw up an entire carton of animal cookies on Mom's freshly scrubbed kitchen floor.

In time, the unfortunate plight of children without mommies and daddies made way for far more pressing concerns, like the travesty of pre-empting my morning cartoons with the lamest parade I have ever seen, the funeral procession for an assassinated president. A year later, Ed Sullivan favoured a terrifying quartet of young British popstars over the appearance of Señor Wences, the one performer that made Ed Sullivan worth watching. As I grew older these events took on greater importance. But neither of those televised events sideswiped me with such jarring profundity — although I wouldn't have recognized it as such then — as the night I stumbled upon Dad watching a German film that I would later learn was Fritz Lang's *M*.

I was busily moving mounds of imaginary earth from one place to another, pushing my dump truck along the hallway that divided the living room from the kitchen, when I heard someone call for "Elsie."

The voice meant nothing but the name, *Elsie*, snapped me out from under the spell of my play. The voice was urgent, distressed, but distant, as though it were calling not just from far away but from another realm, as though part of dream or a memory.

Elsie. Achingly familiar. Instinctual.

I walked into the living room, where the voice seemed loudest — a woman's voice, her accent thick with concern.

Elsie, the name dangling on the edge of my memory as familiar as if it were my own. The image of someone — maybe Elsie, herself — rushed through my thoughts, but the picture didn't stay long enough to be observed. I stood beside my dad's chair. Dad never watched television alone unless it was a hockey game.

"Where's Elsie?" I asked, though, under the circumstances, it was not the question I needed answered. I needed an answer to "Who's Elsie?"

"There," Dad said, nodding toward the screen as though there were no divide between television and living room. Elsie could at any moment step out of her black-and-white world and into ours.

I looked at the screen of the television to see a frightened-looking round-faced man with eyes as large as Ping-Pong balls take a little girl's hand, buy her a balloon, and lead her away so that she was never to be seen again. The words they spoke were unfamiliar, and I was too young to decipher the letters that appeared at the bottom of the screen.

"They're speaking German," Dad said. Dad didn't need to read the words appearing at the bottom of the screen. His parents spoke German. He understood German. Which should've meant, or so I thought, that I could understand and speak German, too.

"Did that man hurt that little girl?" I asked, hoping Dad would tell me that the little girl went to her friend's house and would soon be back with her mother.

"Looks that way," Dad said, his response more reflex than reflective. I couldn't have been more than an interruption in Dad's head.

"Is she dead?"

"I imagine so."

"Why?" The concept of a child's death, particularly their murder, filled me with a new dread.

"Who knows what makes people do what they do," said Dad. His distance from me made the film seem even more frightening than it was, yet I couldn't leave. I had to know more about the frightened man. I had to know if the little girl reappeared. I had to know why the terrified man cowered in a basement.

"Why's he crying?" It didn't seem right to me that a man capable of hurting a child could also be capable of tears.

"Because it's not his fault. He can't help who he is."

I considered Dad's answer, not fully understanding but nonetheless feeling that there is, in this world, a chance of uncontrolled violence.

"Could he hurt me?" I asked.

Dad didn't answer right away. He waited, maybe to consider what would be an appropriate answer to reassure a four-year-old that the world wasn't a randomly dangerous place where children could be lured by balloons never to be seen again. Or perhaps he was waiting for a break in the film's action.

"It's a movie," he finally said.

Had I been open to the messages the universe was sending out, I might have recognized that it wasn't just a movie. It was a trigger to something in the past, and a warning about the future.

* * *

The way Mom told the story you'd think they adopted the baby Jesus. I didn't mind; there was a reverential and mystical quality to her telling that suited me just fine. Her voice shifted a few octaves, losing the sharp, no-nonsense edge so common, I think, in people raised in the Depression era. It was a voice suited to a favourite childhood bedtime tale full of magic and wonder recited not from the heart but of the heart. Uncle Bob said that was the Irish in her. "The Irish are natural storytellers, and your mom was a Flaherty long before she was an Ernst. Remember that," he told me.

It was best to wait until Mom was comfortable in her armchair and had picked up her knitting. The needles would dance at a master's clip, the wool rising in an endless thread from a bag sitting on the floor beside the chair.

I sat at the end of the couch closest to her chair. There I watched as she looped tiny rings of wool from one needle to the other, listening to the tips of the needles strike a musical *click, click, click,* like a distress signal from a forest insect. The repetition of knit one, purl two was hypnotic enough to clear her head after a day's worth of doing busy chores about the house.

In the corner of the room, a birdcage rattled with the movements of a song-less canary, ironically named Tweety, hopping from perch to perch. At our feet, our dog, Clancy, getting on in years, stretched on the floor, elongating her body to the length of a fair-sized rug, the bottom of her greying snout pressed against the carpet, her eyes staring sleepily ahead. From outside came the distinct sound of an engine decelerating as a vehicle veered from highway asphalt to gravel shoulder — a pickup truck turning onto the lane that ran along the length of our property down to Montag's farm, its headlights bouncing in synchronized rhythm over the ruts, crunching gravel like crushed ice beneath the weight of its wheels. Something heavy and metallic, a loose toolbox perhaps, bounced in the truck's bed, sending out a crash of steel against steel, creating what Mom called *quite the racket.*

"You're going to lose it if you don't tie it down," Mom said, always quick to offer advice to those who neither wanted it nor heard it.

"Mom?"

"What now?" Mom's response had the lament of someone waiting to be asked to lend money.

"Tell me about how you decided to adopt me."

"What do you mean, how we decided?"

Telling the adoption story, or any of her stories, whether it was the ghost in the rocking chair or the angel outside her bedroom window, required a perception of humility. My role was to beg her to tell the story; her role was to resist and present the illusion of disinterest.

"You know, when you decided."

She responded with an exaggerated sigh, flushed with full-on irritation as if telling the story required her to leap from her chair and dance a jig across the room.

"Haven't you heard that story enough?" she asked.

And I'd say, "No, I haven't."

Mom put on an impressive show about how she must have told the story umpteen billion times, and can't she have a moment of peace to herself? It was a show designed to downplay any notion that she took any personal pleasure in having an audience. I didn't mind, except that it seemed like an awful waste of time since she would tell the story, anyway. And, as expected, she sighed once more for good measure, sat back, focused on her knitting, and began the story.

It started at the Harmony Lunch diner.

"You sauntered in like you owned the place." Mom took a break from her knitting and did a little pump with her arms, mimicking a younger me in a jaunty gait. Mom preferred to create visuals with broad pantomimes and caricatures rather than with words. I'd see myself at three, stepping into a diner, quite likely my first, with an assertiveness fuelled by naïveté and innocence. I'm a little man, enthusiastic and curious but dignified. I didn't buy the *jaunty gait* shtick, which I found vaguely insulting.

"We took you in for ice cream. It was me, your dad, and Anna."

"And Valerie?"

"I don't know where Valerie was — off gallivanting somewhere. You know teenagers."

I didn't, of course, but recognized that being a teenager was explanation enough for all sorts of weird behaviours.

"Do you want to hear the rest of the story or not?" she asked.

I did.

"You marched in, made a beeline for the counter, and tried climbing up on the stools. You would have fallen off and cracked your skull open if I hadn't been there. We tried to get you to sit in one of the booths, but you'd have none of that. It had to be those stools because they spun, you know."

"I was spinning around on the stool?" I asked, not really a question but a reminder to not leave out any details (especially any detail that would highlight my more winsome attributes).

"Well, you wanted to. I don't know if we let you or not. Probably not."

"But you let me sit on them."

"You weren't going to have it any other way. I thought to myself, if he falls off, serves him right, he'll know better next time. But, of course, I was there to make sure you didn't."

"I remember."

"Don't know how you can."

"I remember sitting on the stool at the counter, and we ordered ice cream."

"Right. And you had to have yours in a bowl to make soup out of it."

Admittedly, the ice-cream-into-soup memory was familiar but only in a foggy, dream-like way: sitting at that counter, making soup by mashing up the ice cream until it melted into a cool, sweet, liquid pool. I saw my mother sitting beside me. My mother, who, with a knowing and slightly patronizing wink in her voice, the kind that adults exchange when accommodating the silly whims of a child, told the waitress, a faceless young woman who carried with her an aura of apathy, that I required a bowl, adding, in abstract intonation, "*So he can make soup out of it, don't you know.*"

The memory is fuzzy; a flash from a drama played in a constant loop without the benefit of colour or definition, the picture marred by static and poor reception. I see myself on the stool, little pants, little shirt, little shoes, brush cut. I'm a silent witness to my own past, like Alastair Sim in *A Christmas Carol*, an observer without influence. But once Mom neared the end of the story, the memory belonged only to her.

"I got you down from the stool, and you made a beeline for your father and took his hand, just like that. No one was telling you to do it. You just did it. Like it was the most natural thing in the world. And that's when we knew you were ours." Mom said all this without looking up from her knitting.

And the adoption story ends on a pictorial image of an orphan taking the hand of the one person willing to provide him with a family and a home. Rockwell could not have sketched it better.

But it's in that exact moment that an orphaned child ran across the floor of the Harmony Lunch diner and took the hand of the one person who would do him the most harm.

I trust what Mom told me about that day was true. The understanding of my history relies on it. But, if her version is accurate, if her memory is correct, if I did take my dad's hand and, by doing so, sealed my fate forever, then I only have myself to blame. There is no other recourse.

Chapter 6

- - - - - - - - -

Sounds from the kitchen — the opening of cupboard doors, the clinking of a coffee cup removed from the shelf, the popping up of toast from the toaster — allowed me the fantasy that the night before never happened. Maybe it didn't. Maybe it was a one-off, a fluke to never be repeated.

Reinforced on the strength of this hope, I struggled out of bed. I went downstairs into the washroom, stared at myself in the mirror, and wondered why I couldn't see my face anymore. There was the reflection of a weaker, lesser me. This was the face I was about to show to my dad. A face that grinned though scarred in sin and sickness. If I was about to embark into a game of ignorance, then this was going to be my game face.

In the mirror I saw behind me the Wild Boy from my room. Smirking, I imagine, at how pitiful I was being. But what was done was done. There would be no unravelling the mess of humiliation I woke up in. My hope that it had been a dream was crushed under a weight of shame. The only thing left to do was to start the business of forgetting — an effort that would have to last until one of us, or both of us, were dead. How many years, then, until I was in the clear? Eighty, maybe seventy — with some luck, sixty — years of living with this secret. The Wild Boy laughed and whispered that there was no chance of keeping the secret. But I thought I could do it — pretend to be alive for sixty years. Others have done more with worse. And so, I did what they did in the movies when people stood in front of mirrors asking questions that couldn't be answered: I ran the faucet and splashed cold water across my face. But the Wild Boy laughed even harder because he knew that would do nothing. And he was right.

I braced myself for the first encounter with Dad since the weirdness of the night before. I looked to him for clues on ways to act, but his world hadn't changed. How could that be? I was stuck in the insanity of the night before, surviving on a determination to live a lie, despite an unforgiving power of guilt.

"No one needs to know. It'll be our secret," is the only thing he said as I left the house to catch the school bus. This is how I knew he forgave me and that he was going to protect me from anyone discovering my shameful behaviour.

* * *

The school bus picked me up at the foot of Chapman's driveway. I filled every moment of silence, no matter how brief, no matter how fleeting, chattering not talking, about the good things, staying up all night, about having chips and pop whenever I wanted, about Dad taking me to the drive-in on the weekend. Paul, Scott, Carol, Neil, and Marianne stared at me like I was a television that's been left on.

The bus was more than half-full when it reached us. Brad and Dennis sat near the back with one seat saved for me and another seat saved for Terry, who would get on board at the next stop. Seating on the bus was arbitrary, although preferred seats were established and adhered to by the end of the first week. Dennis always controlled the conversation, but that day I took over. I repeated everything I told the kids at the bus stop, about staying up late and how I wasn't even tired! And that I watched *Rowan & Martin's Laugh-In* and *Bonanza* and even *The Tonight Show Starring Johnny Carson*.

"I hate *Bonanza*," Dennis said, but his dismissal didn't have the same bite that it would have were I not stoked on anxiety and adrenalin.

"There's an all-night Clint Eastwood Man with No Name marathon at the drive-in this weekend. Dad's taking me." There was no way Dennis could disrespect "The Man with No Name."

"I've already seen them," said Dennis. "In a real theatre. You can't see the movie properly at drive-ins, plus you're distracted by all the cars and the sound is awful." Thing is, Dennis's parents never went to the drive-in, so I don't know if he'd ever been.

Terry got on the bus and took the seat in front of Dennis.

"My dad has a book about people having sex and it describes exactly how they do it," I blurted out, before the Clint Eastwood movie marathon had time to settle in their minds.

"Are there pictures?" Terry asked.

"*Northwest Passion*," I said.

"What?"

"That's the name of the book, *Northwest Passion*."

"My brother has plenty of those kinds of books with pictures," said Dennis. He almost succeeded in derailing attention from me onto to him, but I still held the winning card.

"There's a part in the book where two girls kiss and touch each other in a car." The noise from the other kids on the bus covered up most of what I said, not that I was being particularly careful.

Terry, Brad, and Dennis were speechless. Until …

"Two girls?" This was Terry.

"So, what, you go snooping around in your parents' room looking for dirty books?" I don't imagine Dennis being pleased at how I gained Terry's attention. It amounted to a form of mutiny.

"My dad showed me. He let me read it."

There was some skepticism as to the validity of whether *Northwest Passion* existed and even more skepticism as to whether my dad let me read it, but the skepticism sank beneath my unquestionable certainty that it was true. I kept talking, bringing up bits and pieces of *Northwest Passion*, describing the colour art on the softcover jacket depicting the big stocky woodsmen whooping it up in a cabin with barely dressed and highly agreeable women. I held their attention for the entire bus ride. Even Dennis had to listen. By the time we got to Baden Public School, I'd run out of things to say. I was exhausted and so, it seemed, were Brad, Terry, and Dennis, stunned by the images of naked women and lustful men willing to do anything to each other, even women who touch other women.

That day I was quiet at school. My energy spent. I fell asleep in class. My teacher wanted to know if I would like to lie down in the nurse's office. I did. No one questioned why I might be so tired. I suppose they thought I had been up all night worrying about my mother.

Dad was home when I returned. He asked me if I told anyone about last night. I told him I didn't. He said, good, because people wouldn't understand. Then I asked about Mom, and he said that she's doing as well as could be expected.

After dinner, I went out to play with Doug. We passed an hour or two riding bikes in our driveway — a paved area that seemed to our young eyes to be the size of a small runway. We imagined ourselves to be Steve McQueen and Charles Bronson in *The Great Escape* on stunt motorcycles. Then we ditched the bikes and went into the backyard, standing up on the swings pretending to be superheroes flying to someone's rescue, leaping from the swings and landing on our feet, standing in heroic defiance against whatever evils we decided were worth the battle.

We always won.

The evening wore down, and it was time to go home. Doug went to his houseful of brothers.

If I didn't much like being an only child before, I liked it even less with Mom gone.

I went into the house without being called, doubting that Dad's parental skills would even consider that it was starting to get dark, and I should be home. Dad was on the couch on the opposite side of the room facing the television screen. I went into the front room, laid on the floor, and watched the screen. I was in my pyjamas. The night before faded away. I began to feel safe again.

Until …

"You couldn't be comfortable down there," Dad said.

"I'm fine."

"You shouldn't be lying on the floor. You'll catch a cold." A new tactic. A parental tactic. A captain without credentials commanding the crew, "Come, lie on the couch with me."

"I don't want to be tickled," I said, laughing. Letting him know that I realized it was all just a game — like a naughty joke kids tell each other in the playground.

"No tickling, I promise," Dad said.

Deciding what's right and wrong was my father's job. I didn't know how to disobey. It was inconceivable to me that my father would do me harm. He was a father who simply wanted to embrace his son. A father who wanted to be playful, interactive, affectionate. A friendship was forming between me and this man who spent too much time working on his yard. A man who recognized me but who rarely saw me. A man who knew me by name but not by heart. He called me over. Kindly. Offered me a place with him on the couch. I laid down in front of him, the two of us parallel on the couch, me facing the television. A father and his young son. Then his hand moved onto my stomach, holding me in place. He didn't want me to fall off the couch, he said.

Then his hand moved again. So slowly that I wasn't sure if it was moving at all. I laid quietly. I was still. I stared at the television trying not to feel his fingertips working their way beneath the waist band of my pyjamas, inching down until he had me in his hand. This time it didn't tickle. So, I suppose, in an obscure, tilted manner, Dad kept his promise.

Chapter 7

- - - - - - - - - -

I could never impress Doug with stories of my adoption no matter how many lies I told to make things more interesting. Doug could not be convinced that Clint Eastwood, James Bond, or even Bobby Orr (which at least had a shot at being true) was my real dad. He referred to my adoption as my Hallmark moment, and I hardly needed to know what a Hallmark moment was to know he was being disrespectful.

"You're just jealous that you're not adopted," I shot back.

"You're just jealous that you don't have glasses," Doug said.

And with that we were even.

We'd been on foot since ditching our bikes in a sheltered hollow at the base of a wooden bridge behind Montag's farm that arched above the railway tracks. The Montags were just about the oldest people we knew. Mrs. Montag dressed like the women did in western movies who settled in farmhouses and rode in covered wagons. She had wire-framed glasses, and her cheeks were so rosy as to seem unreal. I thought she looked like Mrs. Wilson from my *Dennis the Menace* comics. Once Doug and I asked Mrs. Montag if she'd be our grandmother because neither of us had grandparents, but we didn't ask Mr. Montag to be our grandfather because he had no front teeth, and when he grinned, he showed off a gaping row of uneven pink flesh as if the inside of his mouth was stuffed and shaped with wads of chewed-up bubble gum.

Doug and I were convinced that the Montags' house was haunted. Doug ought to know, what with the late-night horror films, scary comics, and *The Twilight Zone* series. Doug said the shutters on a haunted house are always broken and dangling from the windows, the chimney will look as if it's ready to crumble, and the outside walls are covered in veins of dried-up vines. Haunted houses are also surrounded by trees that are dead or dying and with branches that bend and twist into witches' fingers that point toward the house and dare you to go inside.

We were following a trail already embedded into a forest floor made of pine needles and hard earth, trampled from the weight of travellers who took a path of least resistance around roots and toppled logs, passing moss-covered rocks, along patches of fern and wild flowers and the chance of poison ivy, between tree trunks and above the swampy pools of mud where frogs and turtles sat camouflaged amongst the decaying leaves and fallen branches, and garter snakes wove between the bulrushes, sensing the possibility of dinner on the tip of their tongues. We walked farther along the forest trail. Doug found a branch large enough to thrash against the weeds that dared to cover our path.

"Hallmark makes those cards you get on birthdays that are supposed to make you feel good, but they're just corny," he said, hacking the tops off a wayward patch of milkweed.

"I know what a Hallmark moment is." I gave him my best who-in-hell-doesn't-know-what-a-Hallmark-moment-is look before beginning a search for a branch of my own.

In time we needed a place to sit, the lure of an unheard siren song daring us to linger in the forest longer than we intended. We found a rock large enough for the two of us to rest. We drank from our canteens, an essential accessory on adventures and hikes, recently filled with the cold run of water that we shared with the cows out of the moss-lined trough. For a while nothing was said, or if there was, I would have been doing the talking. Doug stared at his feet, drawing lines in the ground with a stick.

And then:

"What's with your dad?" Doug asked, his eyes watching the progress of the troughs he was digging. As much as I hoped he meant Bobby Orr, I could be pretty sure that he didn't. A few days back, Doug had seen something he wasn't meant to see. I knew even then that he saw it, but until that moment, we were both pretty good at pretending nothing happened.

Doug had been my best friend since moving from our home in Waterloo on Royal Street to Waldau Crescent, a small community of perhaps twenty houses, mostly farmland with spotted patches of forests between the fields, that everyone called Petersburg. Mom had sold the move from Waterloo to Petersburg on the argument that there was plenty of room for Clancy to run free and all sorts of trouble for me to get into. Because apparently country trouble is more wholesome than city trouble.

"How do you mean?" I asked, but Doug didn't answer. I wondered if he even knew he asked it, like it was a thought that he never meant to say aloud. Something at the end of the stick — once a machete, now an efficient tool for boring holes and dragging trenches in the dirt — demanded his attention. He poked the stick farther into the dirt, prodding at an insect-shaped clump of something. Then he withdrew the stick and leaned in closer, but there was nothing to see except the churned-up remains of a decomposed leaf or a chip of rotting bark slowly returning to the earth.

It didn't matter. I knew exactly what he meant.

* * *

It had been an unusually hot day.

Doug said, "The heat today is stagnant."

And I said, "It sure is."

And he said, "You don't even know what stagnant means."

And I didn't bother to even try to answer because I knew he was going to tell me, anyway. He wouldn't have been able to help himself.

"Stagnant means that the heat sort of just hangs there doing nothing, and it makes you even hotter than you should be."

"I know."

"Then use it in a sentence."

And I said, "What, are we in school or something?"

Doug thought the heat would be less stagnant in the bush behind Montag's farm because of the shade, so I went into the house to tell Dad that Doug and I were going to the bush because the heat's too stagnant up here. And Dad, who was sitting at the kitchen table working on a crossword puzzle, looked at me with a look filled with disgust.

"Why you telling me? Why should I care what you do?" he said, and I wondered what I did to offend him, but only long enough to get out of the house, hop on my bike, and madly pedal away from there.

I stayed well ahead of Doug, putting as much distance as possible between me and the morning, down past the shadowy dark garden, the most-likely-to-be-haunted house, along the gravel lane, flinging dust and pebbles out from beneath my tires, riding at full speed beyond the barn to the end of the field where the cows' water trough sat filled with the coldest, clearest, purest spring water we'd ever tasted (it tasted even better when the cows drank alongside us), plus a blue block of salt called a cow lick that we broke pieces off of, knowing full well that it was called a cow lick for good rea-son. We rested when we reached the bridge, dropped our bikes at the top of the arch, and sat with our legs dangling over the side, hoping we had timed it so the train would pass below and we could imagine we were Robert Conrad and Ross Martin from *The Wild Wild West* jumping off the bridge and on top of the passing freight cars chasing a villain along the top of a moving locomotive. But after fifteen minutes of staring down the long stretch of iron rails and idly speculating how much weight the bridge could take before collapsing, we got up and continued on our way, down the dirt lane to where that path narrowed and trailed off into a footpath that disappeared into the forest.

The stagnant heat got a slight push from an afternoon breeze across a field dotted with the butter-yellow tops of dandelions whose heads waited to puff into cottony clouds of seedlings ready to be tossed by an even stronger wind or plucked and set to flight on the whispers of someone's wish. Beneath our feet the velvet spurs from green thistles lay close to the ground almost hidden, yet we still stepped aside as if they had the capacity to stretch out their thorns and stab us in the ankles.

We stepped from the fields into instant dusk. The forest's magic was to alter all perspective: sight, sound, touch, and smell. The strength of the afternoon sun was crushed by crowds of towering pines and maples, shading the forest floor in an overcast of crimson-filtered hues. The forest was in a constant state of disarray that shifted and changed so that nothing remained familiar regardless of how often we'd returned to the same spot: footpaths that once curved left now curved right, fallen trees had rotted away or had been replaced by pockmarks of fungi and moss, new trees sprouted from damp piles of decayed leaves, and a fresh blanket of pine nee-dles and wildflowers always carpeted the ground. Sound, too, had changed, the hum of cicadas muffled between pillars of cedars and pine while the hidden lives of inner-forest residents — frogs and insects, salamanders and snakes, squirrels and chipmunks — went about the business of maintaining the ecosystem. We caught a frog, held it in our hands, then released it back into the swamp. For a few hours I forgot the heat and the stagnant feelings collected from the things that happened this morning and over the past two weeks, things that were not going to happen ever again because Mom was coming home tomorrow.

I looked forward to being eight again where the biggest issue I had to deal with was how to trap a frog without getting a soaker or being startled by stepping too close to a snake. Eventually, the heat, even among the shade of these trees, became too much. What we needed was to dive into a clean, cool pool of water.

The Chapmans had a pool, but I was not allowed to ask if I could go swimming, not even during the "neighbourhood" hour. I had to wait for an invitation. And so, I stood with Doug inside the fenced-in pool watching the other kids frolic in the water, leaping from the sides of the pool and off the diving board.

I felt I chatted up Mrs. Chapman quite nicely. She was lounging in a deck chair still alert to the kids in the water. I'm not sure how she managed it — all those kids running amuck in their pool. They even built girls' and boys' change rooms by the side of their house. I talked to Mrs. Chapman about the weather, how hot it is, how nice it is to have a pool to cool off in, how kind it is of her to set aside an hour each day to let the neighbourhood kids swim: "My that is nice of you, not so many people would be so generous"; but Mrs. Chapman was too focused on the safety of her guests to pay me much attention. Doug wasn't much help; he was just nodding his head and agreeing with everything I said. "Boy, it sure has been hot lately." "No question, that water does look refreshing." "Sure is nice to have someone in the neighbourhood with a pool — particularly someone so generous with it."

Our efforts were lost in a muddle of children in bathing suits having fun. Finally, I pulled out my trump card. A message so clear it was impossible to miss and yet still maintained the rule my parents had set — that I must be invited.

"You know," I said to Mrs. Chapman, "my parents say I can't ask to go swimming. I have to wait to be invited."

Mrs. Chapman looked at me and smiled. "Well then, would you like to go swimming?"

As I ran home dragging Doug with me to get my bathing suit and my dad's permission, I heard Mrs. Chapman laugh and say, "Well, that's a roundabout way to not ask if you could go swimming."

So, it was my fault when I'm sent scurrying along the floor, struggling to get my balance and get out of my father's range, the floor turning into a pool of oil sending my feet slipping out from under me, the muscles in my legs collapsing. Because I asked to go swimming. Dad fell into a rage, sucker-swiping (wasn't quite a punch) me with the back of his hand, sending me sprawling into the hallway. Because I asked to go swimming? Or because I preferred swimming over grabbing every opportunity to spend alone time with him. My crime was not acknowledging the routine that had been set up, ignoring the father-son ritual that was established.

And so, my father reacted out of pain and jealousy.

Until that moment, I had not known my dad to be violent. His attack was spectacular — a manic attack as wild and unstoppable as any barroom brawl I'd seen in a western or cop drama. Dad jumped out of the kitchen chair, shoving it across the kitchen floor so Clancy had to get up and move out of its way. Dad rose like the dead rising from the earth. A ferocious ape released from its cage, swinging his arms at me, knocking me across the face with a force that sent me against the wall in a hallway so narrow I ricocheted off one side and back again against the other, and when I hit the floor and became too low for his arms to reach me, he started to kick. But the hallway was narrow, preventing him from getting much momentum with his legs.

I was limp, unresisting, dazzled by his amazing display of brutish, uncontrollable hostility. I was learning new things about Dad every day. Even as I cowered, as I tried to run, this latest discovery into my dad's psyche fascinated me. His movements weren't fluid; they were heavy and erratic. He had trouble holding on to me, keeping me where he needed me to be to get in a proper swing. I wasn't ducking the blows, I was merely slipping away from them.

I had learned to deal with Dad's advances — gave in to his whims that allowed me to be stripped naked, fondled, pressed up against, and manipulated so that my hands and my body, by the nature of my complicity, fulfilled whatever desire took over him. Yet as much as I submitted, I still withheld, hoping to limit any physical harm and to preserve a minuscule amount of dignity. I had guidelines that, if I granted Dad most of his demands, I could miraculously get away with not performing others. But this was new. I didn't see Dad's sexual attacks as violent — not then — this was different. This was frightening. This I needed to escape. I would have to rethink my survival strategy to include beatings.

I heard the Wild Boy, a shocked response of *Whoa!* that sounded close to admiration. And then I felt him trying to pull me to my feet. But the Wild Boy couldn't get a proper grip. My legs pumped helplessly against the floor like pistons pushing to start an engine. My hands managed better traction, so I was able to drag myself down the hall and to the bottom of the stairwell. Only then could I make my escape, first in a backward crab walk, dodging his feet before finding a footing so I could turn around and scramble on all fours up the stairs and into my room.

In my room, I fell onto the bed — crying, if I wasn't too shocked to do so. The Wild Boy sat beside me.

Well, said the Wild Boy, *looks like the honeymoon's over.*

Doug sat outside the kitchen door waiting for me on the front steps. He waited while I went in to ask my father if it was all right if I could, on this hot and humid summer afternoon, go swimming at the Chapmans' pool. Doug didn't run when he heard the commotion inside. He didn't move. Doug sat on the steps, frozen, his head down, trying to believe that nothing was wrong.

The blind laws of obedience — like a falling rock obeying the law of gravity, or a wild animal bending to instinct, or a soldier following the rules of engagement. A son is to be obedient to his father. By bringing Doug along I was able to pre-empt all other activities. That wasn't playing by Dad's rules. And so, I paid for that bit of disobedience. Another level of danger had been uncovered, and again I was at fault. Had I not asked to go swimming, this wouldn't have happened. Had I done what was expected, told Doug to go home, pretended that I could change into my bathing suit without incident, then I could have avoided this outburst. But the Wild Boy, moved in the aftermath of Dad's fury by uncharacteristic empathy, questioned why I thought things would be different.

Would it matter what you were doing? he asked. *Had you been writing, would he not come into your room, lie on your bed, and ask what your story is about? And what would you do? You'd be thrilled, forgetting what happened the last time he showed interest. And then what? He'd ask you to read. And you would, believing he was truly interested, even while you struggled to ignore the hand on your thigh. Nope. The only difference is that this kind of violence is less confusing.*

I heard my father come up the stairs, bracing myself for whatever was to come. But why bother, asked the Wild Boy, *Whatever is to happen will happen.* But Dad's anger was gone. He was calm. Sad. I saw regret in his face, and it took over his entire body — the way he moved, the way he stood, the way he held his head. He stood in the doorway.

"I'm sorry. That shouldn't have happened," he said, considering his hands — the international pose of the forlorn, the guilty, and the ashamed. He was not unlike a child himself, weak and pained and in search of forgiveness. I felt sorry for him. "I shouldn't lose my temper like that. It won't happen again."

"That's okay," was the first and only thing that came to mind.

"You can go swimming. Just don't tell your mother about this, okay?" The things I was not to tell Mom were starting to pile up.

I waited until Dad left my room before changing into my bathing suit — I had learned it was best that way. When I came downstairs, Doug was still waiting on the front steps. It was summer, the front door was open. It wasn't likely that he missed what happened. Still, I left the house, excited to go swimming, announcing, "Let's go!"

"What's wrong with your dad?" Doug said.

Had the forest not stepped in to distract us, or if I were better equipped to find the word that I needed, I might have said something other than "he's excited about Mom coming home."

We poked at dead leaves and rummaged through dirt and said nothing more about it. I think that the forest took it upon itself to shut us down. Whatever thoughts and concerns Doug had about my dad disintegrated and crumbled into a dust that drifted then settled on the forest floor, never to be talked about again.

There was still one more night before Mom got home.

"Just one more session," Dad said.

Christ, how I wished he wouldn't call it that. *Sessions.* That's the name Dad came up with to call that thing we did when he thought no one was looking. My stomach churned just to hear him say it; I suppose because I knew what it meant, and more so, because I knew what was to follow. Our sessions. An arrangement so heinously personal that it could only be referenced in vague, clinical words. Our sessions: like a regrettable necessity, a physical examination or intimate and invasive study where I ended up naked and submissive.

He'd catch me at the bottom of the stairs. He never missed an opportunity.

"How about a quick session?" he'd say, but it wasn't a question. It was never a question. Translated, "how about" meant "we are about to have." And no matter how long the sessions were or weren't, they were never quick. "Last time," he'd add, his smile morphing into a foolish pout he could have stolen off the face of a coquettish five-year-old. I laughed because to do anything else would be to take this from a naughty little secret to something ugly and dangerous — something that it already was.

"No," I would tell him, and I would tell him again and again and again as if the choice had ever been remotely mine. I would tell him after he'd found me in whatever room I was using to avoid him, or when he had me pinned on the couch, or when he said he was just checking to see if I was doing my homework. He kept at me until I reached a point where my body froze and I could no longer pretend I had the power to disobey (because it's wrong to not do as your father tells you). So, he did what he wanted, and I would let him. I was too weak to say no with the strength and the persistence needed to stop him. Before long, my body began to betray me in ways I never knew a body could. By then we were too far gone to stop. I had stepped off the edge of the Earth and there was no coming back.

"You said the last time it would be the last time."

"I know." He tilted his head, sheepishly implying an impish child-like guilt, a little boy caught in a tiny white lie, like the whole thing was just a kooky habit that was hard to kick — like eating too many cookies before dinner.

"One more session and that's it. We need to stop for sure after this."

He said we need to stop, when what I wanted to hear him say was that *he* needed to stop. But I wasn't about to fuss over pronouns, especially since I knew Mom would soon be home and things would return to normal.

But the Wild Boy wouldn't stay silent. His voice grew louder and more frequent. He couldn't leave things well enough alone. Funny thing is, though, he seemed angrier with me than anything or anyone else.

You *must stop? He means* he *must stop, right? Or no?*

"One more time," Dad repeated, something he'd continue repeating until I eventually complied. Of course I complied; after all, he had been so kind lately. He apologized for being angry. He let me go swimming. What kind of son would I have been if I was not kind in return?

He thinks you're in this together. And then. *Christ, you think so, too.*

The Wild Boy was goading me into action, but action would have been stupid. Why nitpick over who was responsible and who wasn't? Especially when Mom was coming home. It was over. All I had to do was wait out the morning.

Dad stood behind me, firmly gripped my shoulders and man-oeuvred me down the hallway like I was a push toy being turned left, then right, in a steady and constant momentum that kept my feet shuffling forward. I was not so much led but pushed up the stairs. Whether we turned left into my room or right into my parents' room was his discretion. It was his only discretion. All that mattered was that I be the doll for him to play with. He decided we were to use his room — their room, the room, and the bed he and Mom would later be sharing. He laid me on their bed where I stayed, still, while his fingers danced over me as though he were playing an instrument, but unlike his keyboard or the Hawaiian guitar, I refused him the courtesy of a song. Dad read the silence as evidence of my consent.

Mom had been gone two weeks, and in that time, Dad had crammed in as many sessions as possible: before school, after school, just before bedtime, and if enough time had lapsed between the time I had gone to bed and the time he was ready to call it a night, he'd wake me for "a night-cap session." Each session began and ended with a promise that "this would be the last time." But with Mom coming home, he had no choice.

So, on the morning of the day before Mom was to return, Dad once again said, "Just one more time," and again, I said, "Okay, but this is the last time. Promise?"

Again, he promised. Again, I believed him. I believed him because of an unspoken oath between a father and his son that a father's promise is sacred. It cannot be broken. To have doubted him would have been cruel. But perhaps the oath doesn't apply to fathers whose sons are adopted.

"But since it's our last time, we should make it special."

Later, when his face was skewed into a horrifying expression that looked something like hunger and he asked if I was ready but didn't wait for an answer, I was jarred to life as if waking from a restless sleep into the middle of a nightmare.

"*No!*" someone yelled. A voice. Not mine, although, at first, I couldn't be sure that I wasn't responsible, except that the voice was stronger than my own. A *no* filled with an undeniable force. Unmistakable. Clear.

It was the Wild Boy. And though I wouldn't have thought the Wild Boy capable of fear, there was in his voice something that sounded like terror. I was jolted into the present. I thought nothing of choices, or resistance or consequences, I thought only to respond to the Wild Boy's cry. A war cry as significant as though it were a call to battle. I put out my hands to ward off an attack. My hands on the top of his head, the only physical contact I ever initiated, pushed back with any strength I could muster, shielding myself from being devoured.

But Dad brushed my hands away as if they were nothing more than fallen leaves.

"It's too late now," he said and closed his eyes, bent his head forward and it was my fault because I shouldn't have waited for the Wild Boy to take charge. I should have said no sooner. And you couldn't just change your mind whenever you felt like it. Those were the rules.

When it was over, I got dressed and went out to play. The world didn't end. And it wouldn't end if I kept the secret. A sinful secret only becomes a sin if the secret is broken. Mom always said I couldn't keep a secret, but I was going to prove her wrong, no matter the cost.

Chapter 8

Mom came home. For a few weeks a form of normalcy returned. Mom's form of normalcy: proper bedtimes, proper meals, and a watchful eye on how much television was seen. And then there was a new normalcy of guarding the secret that continued between Dad and me. But if Dad had been worried about me talking, he didn't need to be. I would never have told. I feared nothing more than being found out. I wanted only to get through my life without anyone ever finding out what happened. And that's where Dad and I seemed to agree.

"Don't tell anyone. You'll be sent back to the Children's Aid," he had said. "Maybe jail. Our name will be mud." Such a strange expression, *our name will be mud*. I had never heard such a thing before.

"What do you mean?" I asked.

"Mud," Dad replied, as if the answer were obvious. "Dirty. Filthy. Mud."

So, now our sin had a colour. It was the colour of mud. It had a texture. I imagined a dark-brown formless blot on the sidewalk.

A thing pigs wallowed in while the rest of the living world stepped around and avoided. This was who we were — a thing people scraped off from the bottom of their boots.

"Then why are we doing it?" I asked, meaning, why do you make me do it? Dad had led me into something that would be a lifelong shame. We were in this sin together. This was our shame that I carried for both of us. I knew this to be something that I would have to keep from everyone, forever. The sole responsibility I had in life was to never let anyone know. I didn't want my name to be mud.

"Why? Because it feels different," Dad said, as though this were reason enough, "but we have to stop." Spoken as if the idea were his.

"I keep asking to stop, and you keep saying we will, but we don't."

"Well, now we really do have to."

I discovered that the expression *our name will be mud* was not just one of my dad's quirky archaic idioms, like calling pudding custard, or referring to peanut butter as peanut-butter bread. The Wild Boy had a particularly scornful reaction to Dad's blundering vocabulary: *What? Peanut-butter bread? What the fuck is peanut-butter bread? Our name will be mud* came from Dr. Mudd, a physician who treated an injured John Wilkes Booth, not knowing that Booth's injury came as he fled the scene after he assassinated President Abraham Lincoln. Mudd was later tried and convicted as a co-conspirator. Like most things, I discovered this bit of trivia through the movies. This one, a film John Ford directed in 1936 called *The Prisoner of Shark Island*, which purports the innocence of Dr. Mudd. I doubt Dad understood the history behind the phrase *our name will be mud*, but he got the implication right.

It only made sense that our name was already mud. Keeping it a secret didn't stop that. Before, there was no name for what we did. *Sessions* didn't aptly describe it. But now Dad gave it a name. An ugly, filthy name. Mud. It didn't matter how much I bathed, how intensely I scrubbed at the dirt. Mud had seeped too deeply into my skin. Forget bad blood — it's mud that ran through my veins. I sweated, cried, and stank of mud. There was mud in every word I said. Dad had given me a name for the rest of my life, and I was forced to conceal my real identity — me as this wicked, disastrous, muddy child. But, in the mire and muck of this secret came a miracle. Patty and Al. I couldn't feel muddy when I was with Patty and Al.

* * *

Mom asked if I wanted to spend the day with Patty and Al. She hadn't been home long, and I think now that the sudden arrival of Patty and Al might have been to give Mom time to rest. Good fortune came so randomly and unexpectedly that I never thought to consider *why*.

"They're going to be picking you up in about an hour," Mom said. I was upstairs, dressed, and back downstairs, sitting on the front stoop waiting for them before Mom had a chance to tell me where they were taking me. This happened a lot that year, whenever news came down that I was to hang out with Patty and Al. I'd often be on the steps waiting, hours before they were scheduled to arrive. Mom thought that was just about the cutest thing I could've done, and she'd tell Patty and Al how I sat there all afternoon, not moving, waiting for them to arrive, and nothing she said could get me to budge. It was more than an hour before they arrived that first time, or if it had been an hour, it was one of those wonky hours that stretched well beyond the frame of its allotted sixty minutes. An hour that lasted so long I feared it wouldn't end until nightfall.

"He sure doesn't wait for his father like that," she added.

"I'm sure that has more to do with the fact that we're going to the CNE than anything else," Patty said. I loved Patty's voice. An unmistakable blend of cheerfulness and curiosity. I think Al felt uncomfortable when Mom said things like that. He responded by stuttering out a few words but never finishing the sentence.

"Oh … now … c'mon … I wouldn't say … I'm sure he … I mean … Don't you, Thom?"

But Mom was right — I'd been spending more time with Patty and Al — I'd have spent every moment of every day with Patty and Al if I could — and it wouldn't have surprised me if Dad felt over-shadowed by this new friendship. Al and Patty were now married. With Al being both a cop and a hockey player and with Patty's barbed humour, they qualified as the most fun couple in our family. Val and Wayne were parents, and so were officially grown-ups, leaving Patty and Al as the new reigning sovereignty with me, their chosen sidekick.

Al and Patty took me everywhere, picking up the slack Dad left behind: stock-car races, baseball games, the drive-in, and Al's hockey games (sports took on a new level of interest when you were a close friend of one of the players, and besides, I'd be with Patty, who could make any occasion fun). But everyone loved Al, even Dad, so I couldn't imagine he would have felt threatened. Then again, there were a lot of things about Dad that I would not have imagined and yet ended up being true.

It was late when we returned from the Exhibition. I went straight to bed, exhausted but filled with the excitement of a full day of amusement rides, carney games, candy floss, and caramel popcorn. I hadn't noticed that Dad wasn't home until Mom woke me up from a deep sleep saying, "Come on, we've got to fetch your stupid arse father."

We hopped into the Rambler, me still in my pyjamas, and drove through the night to a house I'd never been to before.

It was a hell of a night for Dad, piss-dead drunk, looking daft and confused, a freshly risen zombie propped up in a chair at the end of a card table. Three other zombies sat with him, each filling out one side of the card table. Poker-playing zombies who Dad called friends. Had they been playing crazy eights, I might have sat in for a round, but Mom abruptly steered me away from the table. Out of harm's way, according to Mom. I had a perfect view of the table where the drama unfolded, in an alcove that sat between the strange living room and an entranceway that led into a kitchen. There were potato chips on the card table, and I desperately wanted some, but none were offered.

One of the card players called himself Dino, and when I heard the name I laughed because it was the same name as Fred Flintstone's pet dinosaur. But the man called Dino shot me a look that startled me into silence.

We were at a stranger's house. More me than we. I was at a stranger's house. Dad seemed to know this place, and Mom had no trouble driving us here without so much as a glance at the street signs. The woman of the house, an apparition who showed up quickly at the door, mumbled a few words to my mother, none to me, came and went. Curt, bordering on hostile, as though she were blaming us for whatever decency Dad had breached.

Dad's face looked like a man stunned by his own existence, doing his best to dig through a repertoire of male-bonding humour that would relieve him from the anxiety of having his wife show up to tell him to get his stupid arse home.

Turned out that Dino was not named after Fred Flintstone's pet dinosaur, but after Dean Martin, the suave ladies' man with a perpetual martini in hand. Dino wasn't even his real name. He was just a man who was told one too many times that he looked like Dean Martin (which he did), so it became his sole gift to the world.

Mom plunked me down on a couch in an unlit living room and told me to stay put in the same way she would have told Clancy to stay put had she been there. Don't move, don't listen, don't think, and don't see. It was a dangerous room with Dad drunk, with these men unhinged by booze and cigarette smoke and their wolf-pack-infused bravura. Not sitting, as told, was my lone act of defiance. Instead, I rested my rump on the edge of a cushion. I wasn't up to committing to any kind of comfort. There was nothing to distract me from the drama in the next room. I was that kid pictured at the bottom left-hand page of every Dr. Seuss story — the gawking, baffled traveller still in his pyjamas, watching while some absurd circus unfolds before him. I had a clear view of the card table where Dad and his boys performed. The table shone like a set piece making Dad and his buddies look like summer stock actors in some tragic remounting of a Neil Simon play.

I was there but not there; Oliver Twist shoved in the corner, guarded by a one-eyed bull terrier, with Fagin and Bill Sikes casting occasional glances, while Nancy rouses a den of thieves and scoundrels into a distracting chorus of "Oom-Pah-Pah." If only.

Dino walked over to my mother with arms spread open, a slight tilt in his head, the kind of tilt people have when trying to make amends with an old friend they once offended. My mother kept her arms to her side.

"It's me, Maggie. Good old Dino," Dino said, holding out his arms as if an open stance made his features appear more "Dean-Martinish."

"Yep. I remember." Mom took a half-step back.

If Dino noticed my mother's shift away from him, it either didn't register or it didn't matter. His tactics switched. He turned on the sensitive Dino, a caring, furrowed-brow man of empathy and compassion. "Are you feeling better, Maggie? Are you?" he asked. "I hear you had a stint in the hospital."

Dino was on the move again. He had the swagger of a villain in a gangster movie. His arms wrapped around Mom in a Venus flytrap grip closing on its prey. Then he bent her back — *dipped*, it was called — an acrobatic trick of romance done by fancy dancers and movie stars and newlywed grooms who want to make people laugh. Dino was kissing Mom.

Dad looked on, his face dumb and useless, a buffoon, with cards in his hands, staring at his wife being assaulted by a celebrity look-alike. Dad was no alpha male. Dino was. Dad watched like a kid watching his balloon float away. He did nothing.

Mom tried to push Dino off like she was pushing off a Pepsi bottle that's been held to her lips for too long, but unlike a Pepsi bottle, there would be no stopping it with your tongue.

I considered yelling out "Leave my mom alone!" but didn't. What made me think I'd be better at saving her than I was at saving myself? Besides, what if this is just another adult thing that I don't yet understand?

The room felt dangerous. Mom stepped into something she wasn't equipped to deal with and she brought me along. The kiss stopped. Dino seemed to know just how long a kiss takes to leave the women swooning. He let my mother go and seemed surprised to see her back away, wiping her mouth as if forcing back a gag.

"Let's go," she said to Dad.

"Look out, Clare," someone said. "The boss is here." Hardy-har-har.

"Damn right she is, now get your butt in gear." Mom wasn't handing out options. Dad staggered up from the table knocking it with his lap.

"You going to let little Margie push you around?" said Dino, the big man on campus. Mom mumbled something about the lot of them being too stupid to know when they've had enough. The zombies laughed.

The cool night air sobered Dad up enough to weave his way to the front seat, passenger side. I got the back seat on the ride home. Dad looked to the back seat grinning his death-clown grin. It was hard sometimes, on pitch-black nights, to distinguish between my

father's face and the face of the monsters I'm told don't exist. Dad
leaned far enough back so that his fingers reached my knee. How
could it have been so dark that he could do this without Mom
knowing? Mom, who craned her head in the rear-view mirror to
see what was going on, as if she suspected. But she said nothing
and turned her attention back to the road. I moved out of Dad's
reach. He leaned back farther. Mom would not look. I slid over to
the other side of the car, but Dad looked dejected and then familiar
feelings that I both craved and despised stirred inside me. Kill me/
save me/kill me/save me.

*He's not afraid of being caught. Why should you? Let her see. Let
her know. Here's your chance. End this.*

Right. Let her catch us. I shifted closer, leaned into the front
seat as I would if I were trying to hear what the grown-ups were
saying. I stayed there, letting Dad get what he wanted, waiting for
Mom to see. Mom's eyes flashed from the road to the rear-view
mirror. What was she seeing? Why wasn't she saying something? I
leaned back again out of reach.

We reached home. Mom parked the car and sent Dad and me
in the house together. Sent us in alone. It took a long time for her
to park the car; long enough for Dad to come into my room, with
hopes of continuing what was started in the car. He laughed and
dared me to tell him to stop. The back door opened. Mom came
into the house. Mom at the bottom of the stairs. Dad took his hand
away, but not before giving me a look that said that he was on to me
and next time I wouldn't be so lucky. Dad left my room as Mom
climbed the stairs. Dad stumbling and drunk. Mom didn't ask why
he was in my room. The lights turned off and another night ended.

Chapter 9

- - - - - - - - - - -

Wasaga Beach. The weather couldn't have been better, and almost everyone else in southern Ontario must have thought so, too. Valerie, Wayne, Davy, and little Denny, turning three that year (where does the time go?), came with us but took their own car. I wanted to ride with them, but with all of Denny's sand toys plus their cooler, beach chairs, beach towels, and their fancy beach umbrella, there was no room for me. I rode with Mom and Dad. Good thing that everyone was in a great mood, especially Mom, who was never happier than when she was driving somewhere, even if it was nowhere. I wanted Doug to come along, but Mom said this was a family outing. I didn't argue because family outings, when we were all together and no harm could be done, were still the best of times.

The radio was on but, in our car, there were no summer beach songs like there would have been in Wayne and Valerie's car. Our car settled for easy-listening tunes from Perry Como, Andy Williams, and Peggy Lee, and maybe, for a few miles, the distinctive twang of Tammy Wynette, Charley Pride, and Loretta Lynn from a middle-of-the-road country station with an announcer who introduced himself as "Your Ole' Buddy Hoppy from Good Old Elmireee" putting a quaint country spin on the name of his hometown, Elmira.

Mom kept pointing out sights along the way. Cows grazing in a field facing west. "Look at those stupid cows all facing the same way," she'd say. "Wonder what they're looking at." And then a horse in a field standing on its own. "Poor old guy, all by his lonesome." Then two hitchhikers carrying large backpacks. "Sorry. No room."

I occupied myself in the back seat, moving freely from one window to the other looking for the cows and the horse and the hitchhikers with their backpacks. I told Mom that there was plenty of room for the hitchhikers (but maybe not their backpacks), but she said, "Let them walk. It's a nice enough day."

We arrived early, 10:00 a.m., and already the beach was generously spotted with early risers anxious to secure their optimal spot in the sand. The essence of a beach town is immediately familiar no matter what the time of day. The tiny shanty convenience stores with their screen door entrances and shuttered windows were just opening for a day of selling popsicles, ice cream bars, and cold drinks. Along the main street, someone from the downtown discount store pulled out barrels filled with splash toys and Frisbees and water guns and inflatables, next to the higher-end store that sold bathing suits and goggles and wasn't going to open until eleven. We turned off the main drag to follow a sign that pointed to the marina. As we turned onto the side road we could see the expanse of Georgian Bay, a cool, inviting blue that melded beautifully into the sky. Its size breathtaking, impossible to conceptualize, as though the water itself was eternity. We had reached the end of the Earth. I rolled down my window and all that I had come to associate with the beach rushed into the car: the smells and sounds of summer, of warmth from the sun and sand carried in on a cool lake breeze, of

seagulls crying in swarms in the sky and then again as they landed on the docks, a faint smell of fish either caught and brought to
shore or swept up in the tide, all mixed with the scent of coconut
suntan lotion.

The marina looked ancient, a floating accident at the end of a
dock, the kind of shambled wreck we read about in *The Adventures
of Huckleberry Finn* where Joe finds the corpse of Huck's drunk-
en, abusive father, or the makeshift house Dennis described as "a
shanty" from a book he was reading called *The Grapes of Wrath*.
("Sounds like a shack I read about in a Hardy Boys mystery," I said
to Dennis, but Dennis sneered and said that he didn't read Hardy
Boys.)

Standing near the edge of the dock was a Texaco fuel pump in-
accessible to cars, and I realized with some amazement that this was
to fuel the many boats bobbing in the quays stretching out from
the shore in a carefully organized grid. We did not drive into the
marina where the rich people loaded their boats for their summer
cottages but took the road left. Wayne was several cars ahead but
still in sight. Dad was agitated, which always happened at the first
sign of too many people or traffic confusion.

"Why does he have to drive so fast?" Dad complained of Wayne.
"Always has to be way ahead of everybody else. We're supposed to
stick together." I sat in the back seat wondering what it would be
like if, just once, it was our car that was way ahead of everyone else.

The road followed the beach-line. Cars were parked along either
side on gravel shoulders. Traffic moved slowly, partly out of caution,
partly to take in the view, and partly because families like ours were
looking for a place to park. Wayne found a spot first but reserved
it for us by stopping in front of it and signalling as if he was about
to turn in.

"What's he doing?" Dad asked, pulling up behind him. "He's
just sitting there."

"I think he wants you to park," Mom said.

Dad made a quick calculation of the space Wayne reserved for us.

"I couldn't fit in there," he said, but Wayne, having spotted what could potentially be a second open space, pulled away, leaving Dad with no option but to give it a try or lose it forever.

Cars were coming up behind him hungry to snatch the opportunity from him. If he wasn't going to take it, then the next person would, making him the fool for passing up on what could be the last free parking space for miles.

"Oh, Clare. You could park a boat here," Mom said, finding her playful, feisty voice to add to the challenge. "Or you just get out and I'll slide over and show you how it's done."

"Oh, you wouldn't." To my surprise, Dad was open to playing along.

"Oh yes, I would."

"That'll be the day." Dad turned on his signal and began backing into the open space.

"You just watch me," said Mom. "I'll do to you what I did on the golf course."

"Oh no," Dad laughed, which seemed to alleviate the stress of parking in a tight space while under the constant watch of a growing lineup of impatient and frustrated drivers, for Dad perfectly manoeuvred our vehicle into place in one attempt.

"What?" I asked, although I had heard the golf story almost as many times as I had heard the adoption story.

"Haven't I told you this story before? We just got married and your father decides we should go golfing. I couldn't give a hoot about golf, but Jean liked it, so we go with her and Ted. And your dad isn't liking the way I golf. Phooey on him. I told him that if he doesn't keep quiet, I'm going to throw him to the ground and sit on him. He didn't think I could, so I showed him. I took him by one arm, got my leg behind his leg and pushed him right over. He landed flat on his arse and I sat on him, just like I said I would. That taught him. Your Aunt Jean laughed so hard she peed her pants."

We all laughed at the story. This was working up to being a good day.

Val and Wayne walked back to us, Wayne lumbering beneath the weight of beach paraphernalia, Val a few steps ahead carrying an oversized beach bag she had flung over her shoulder and grasping the hand of Denny, who toddled alongside her. David was instructed to get to the side of the road and stay there. I took David's hand.

The beach was crowded with oversized umbrellas popping out of the sand like mushroom-shaped awnings. The sound of voices, laughter, and splashes mingled together, so that if we were to have closed our eyes, we would still know we were at the beach. Finding a decent spot was as hard as finding a decent place to park, but Wayne, once again, managed to navigate us toward an open spot in the sand where we laid out our blankets and arranged the coolers packed with freshly cut watermelon, fruit juices, and sandwiches. Water from the lake rolled in with sizable swells that curled and broke into whitecaps before spreading up along the sandy shore, encouraging younger kids to try balancing on their flutter boards and inflatable rafts. A few others waited for the water swells to hit their peak height before diving straight into them, allowing the wave to carry them back and dump them on shore.

We removed our outer clothes until we stood beach-ready in our bathing suits and sunglasses.

Mom had me slather on suntan lotion, although I couldn't see the point considering I planned on spending all my time in the water. Val did the same for Denny and David. David was finding the lure of the water too much to stand still. Wayne unfolded the lawn chairs and set up the umbrella. Valerie placed yellow inflatable flotation devices on each of Denny's and Davy's tiny arms and inflating them by blowing into an extended plastic valve. Davy allowed for this as it was a sure indication that water was soon to be involved. Denny kept pulling his off.

The set-up was quick. Mom, Dad, and Valerie dropped into their lawn chairs. Mom lay back, saying her standby comment reserved for moments like this — "I wonder what the poor people are doing today?" — because in Mom's world, poor people have no access to the beach and no desire to lie slathered in coconut suntan lotion beneath beach umbrellas. She warned me to stay in sight and to not go out too far in the water; other than that, I was free to plunge into the water, to feel the spectacular sensation of being weightless, riding the swells that popped up like ski moguls and free to proudly display my fearlessness by putting my whole head beneath the surface.

I spent time with Davy where the water rose to no higher than my knees. Wayne never strayed far from his son's side. Denny was in diapers, so he stood watching his brother splash for a while, finding shells and colourful stones to examine, enjoying the cool run of water lapping beneath his feet. Wayne tempted Davy in farther, and Davy was eager to comply, happy to be on this adventure with his dad, holding on to both his hands as they bounced farther into the lake. Denny went back to his mother. I went out deeper, too, entertaining Davy with my aquatic feats — immersing myself completely in the water, diving head-on into the waves, pumping out spurts of water from my hands like those from the spout of a whale — all the while checking to ensure that my efforts were seen and appreciated by those on shore.

Cheerful bits of revelry rose from the beach where my family sat: the melodic lift of my sister's laugh, my mother's gentle nagging to Dad to "not drown yourself, crazy old coot." I turned to see Dad heading away from the lawn chairs and the beach towels and the cooler and making his way toward the water's edge. Wayne saw him, too. My dad, father of two grown married daughters, a grandfather of three (by this time Anna had a daughter of her own), still in fine athletic form, aged only by slightly thinning and greying hair. His pace was assured as he moved across the sand with the trained efficiency of a beach lifeguard, running out into the water, splashing through the shallows, charging into deeper areas and then with arms out in front, hands pointed and folded over top of each other in the shape of an arrowhead, he arched his body and leapt from land and air and into water. He remained submerged long enough for us to appreciate his form and grace. Then, rising out of the lake, he let out a whoop, flipped his head to rid himself of the excess water that ran into his face, blowing the drops away from his mouth.

"Whoa!" he said to the appreciation of the rest of the family. "That's cold."

"Yahoo!" Val yelled from her beach chair. I heard Mom laugh.

"That's the way to do it, Clare," said Wayne, shin deep in the water, holding on to Davy's hands. "Gets warmer the longer you stay in."

"Yeah. It's nice once you're in," Dad agreed. He swam out farther using what I thought of as the perfect Johnny Weissmuller front crawl. Then, in a motion as fluent as the water itself, he submerged a second time, resurfacing closer to where I stood. "Oh, yeah. This is nice."

Closer to the water's edge, a ripple of water rolled up under Davy's chin. He winced but didn't cry. Wayne was on it immediately with laughs and encouragement, showing Davy how fun it was to have the water splash in your face. Davy coughed and spurted and wiped water away from his eyes, nose, and mouth, and then responded with a demand for more. Wayne started pulling Davy by the arms, allowing his legs to lift so that he was gliding along the top. Valerie waded into the water more cautiously than the rest of us. She dropped a beach towel just out of reach of the water's ebb. Around her neck she wore a camera that she kept one hand on as she moved closer to her husband and son, to get, presumably, a good shot of Davy's day at the beach.

"Davy," she called, with the camera held up to her eyes. "Davy, look this way." Davy gave the lens a huge, hammy smile.

I was in deep enough that the water rose to my chest. I moved by hopping along the lake bottom, the occasional wave pushing as high up as my neck. Dad crouched so that only his head was above, keeping the rest of his body warm and submerged. His arms stretched out and back in constant movement as if treading water.

"Dad, watch," I said, waiting for the next swell of water to come and dive, as he had done, with my arms stretched out in front of me, my hands clasped to a point. I swam underwater for as long as I could, my eyes opened to see the lake bottom, and the feet of other swimmers through the greenish hue. I rose, bounced once to make sure I was in shallow enough water to stand, and wiped the water that dripped from my hair onto my face. But Dad was looking elsewhere. "Did you see, Dad?" I shouted. He turned to me.

"Yeah. That was great. Let's see it again."

So, I waited for the next wave to come along. I looked to make sure he was watching. He was. As before, I dived in, imagining myself to be as graceful as a dolphin born to water. When I resurfaced, he was watching.

"Good," he said. "Now do it again and see if you can swim over to me."

He was not so far from me that the challenge was unthinkable. Most of his body he kept below the surface, creating an illusion of depth — when I stood alongside him, I reached to just below his shoulders — but were he to stand, the water would reach chest level. Besides, I could swim, and he'd be there should I need help.

I dived into the water a third time, and for a third time I caught a glimpse of a new world beneath the water's surface. I saw my father's crouched form ahead of me, the fabric from his boxer-shaped bathing suit moving with the current like a flag waving for my attention. I swam below the water's surface, kicking my legs and driving myself forward with great sweeps of my arms. This time I was Tarzan propelling through a jungle swamp of hungry gators and poisonous water snakes. I kept myself underwater until I was at my father's side, then I popped up and stood beside him. The water covered my shoulders. Dad stood up and grabbed me under the arms to make sure that it was not too deep.

"I can stand," I told him.

"Are you sure?"

"Yep."

He let go. I stood on my toes, lifted my arms out of the water holding them in front of me above my shoulders.

"So, you can," he said. "Do you want to really dive in?"

"Yeah. How?"

"Here," Dad said, "turn around." I turned so my back was to him. He crouched in the water, brought his arms down and interlocked his fingers creating a foothold with his hands. "Okay, step into my hands, I'll toss you up, and you dive in."

"Okay." I placed my foot into his cupped hands, and he catapulted me into the air like he were tossing a Scottish pole. I was flying and loving the sensation of being airborne, then crashing into the water. "Again!" I said, moving back to him for more. "Wayne, Valerie," I yelled. "Watch!"

Wayne and Valerie were now on shore. They'd wrapped Davy in a towel and were walking him back to Mom. Both turned to watch.

"Okay," Val said, shielding her eyes from the glare coming off the water. Davy turned to look, too, probably calculating whether what I was doing was enough fun to join.

"Mom, watch!"

Mom waved her hand from the beach chair. "I'm watching," I heard her say.

I stepped into Dad's cupped hands, and once again I was flung into the air and landed safely in the water. I surfaced, hearing Mom, my sister, and Wayne cheering. Davy shivered beneath an oversized towel. I laughed and hopped back to Dad.

"More?" Dad asked as if the request was unreasonable.

"Just a few more," I pleaded.

"Okay," he sighed, "just a few more. But we have to wait for the right wave."

He lowered himself into the water as he did before, but this time, I didn't feel the cupped hands at my feet. I felt my father's hands beneath the water playing at the waistband of my bathing suit while crowds of families splashed around us.

"Hold on. Waiting for the right wave." His hand slipped inside the elastic waistband. Waiting for the right wave, that's what he said. Waiting for the right wave as his hand moved farther down the front of my bathing suit. From the shore, Mom watched and smiled.

* * *

What I feared more than all else was the agonizing possibility of being caught. I worried more about being caught than I did about grades, friendships, or even the abuse. It was no longer reasonable of me to expect that Dad would stop, even though he continued with the promise of "this is the last time." He wasn't going to stop, and no amount of pleading or praying or threatening could change that. My only option was to live through this until the time came that God or nature decided enough was enough. Or until we got caught.

And what then? What happens when we're caught? What thoughts and excuses and manners of disguises would rush to our minds to save us? What lies would we tell to cover the truth even while standing naked and exposed? Who would we blame? Each other? No one? Me?

Dad was becoming increasingly careless about where and when he initiated our sessions: during camping trips with Mom asleep on the other side of the tent trailer, in the car at drive-ins with people walking around us, once at a public shower assuring me that no one was going to walk in moments before someone walked in, at Wasaga Beach, in the middle of the afternoon with Mom, Valerie, Wayne, Davy, and Denny nearby. Yep. The thorn of responsibility had been handed to me: I had to keep his secret for both of us. I'd be keeping the secret for years to come.

Chapter 10

Aiding and abetting. The Wild Boy sat on top of my dresser, propped up like a life-size doll with his feet dangling over the side. He has done this before, crawled up on the dresser, pushed things aside to make room for himself. I've told him he's not supposed to sit there and if Mom were to come into the room and see the mess he left, we'd be in trouble.

But that just made the Wild Boy laugh. *Your Mom doesn't see anything she doesn't want to see.* The Wild Boy didn't care for Mom. He thought she knew more than she let on. But how could she know if no one told her? The Wild Boy climbed down from the dresser, dropping several inches then landing effortless on both feet, steady and solid, making barely a sound. *I forgot. Can't say anything bad about dear old Mom. But* — and it's here that he stopped and looked at me, his head slightly tilted, his hand raised with a finger lifted to assure I knew a point was waiting to be made — *I just don't think you're as good at keeping secrets as you think you are. Aiding and abetting.* He repeated.

I had known the Wild Boy for over two years. We were eight when we met, alone in my room, him sitting on the very same dresser, dangling his feet in the same way (although then his feet dangled farther up from the ground). Now we were ten, with only a few weeks before turning eleven. The Wild Boy had grown, changing in ways that mimicked my own changes.

"What does that mean?"

What?

"Aiding and a bedding?"

Oh. Aiding and abetting. It means helping a criminal. You know, like keeping their secrets for them. The Wild Boy said things that sounded worth saying, but he didn't know nuts about consequences.

"My name would be mud."

The Wild Boy smiled. *Aiding and abetting,* he said again, and then he left for somewhere without saying where he was going.

* * *

A letter appeared in Dear Abby, an advice column that ran daily on the front page of the *Kitchener-Waterloo Record* and in just about every newspaper up and down and across North America. There was a protocol to reading the family paper — rules to when and how it could be read: I was to wait until Dad and then Mom had read the paper before I went at it, disassembling its pages, pulling out the sections like tossing back bedsheets, scouring through the headlines and bylines for the bits and pieces that fed my preadolescent interests. Dad hated reading a paper with the pages already bent and folded and creased and ruffled, but it was only an occasional complaint, so it was only an occasional rule. I had my routine destinations. Comics at the back of section three. A pause in the middle of the classified section to glimpse at *Gasoline Alley,* a nostalgic comic that survived the Depression but had little to offer in the way of current references and ideas. The entertainment section, mostly ads for films at the local theatres made glorious with epic portraits of John Wayne, Gene Hackman, Raquel Welch, Claudia Cardinale, Dustin Hoffman, and other stars, banners with four or five stars and spouting critical praise announcing it to be the funniest or the most powerful or the most thrilling or the best film of the year, and the occasional film review, which I devoured with the same interest most of my peers devoured the sports section. The horoscope, whose advice I was determined to follow but dismissed almost immediately. The Ben Wicks etching on the front page reflecting current events, even though I rarely got the joke, Wicks's political cartoon often featuring the exaggerated features of easy-to-spot political leaders: Diefenbaker, Trudeau, Joe Clark. And then came the Dear Abby column. Every Dear Abby letter popped with tragedy, loss, grief, fights with rowdy neighbours, uncontrollable children, inappropriate friendships, mothers-in-law, ethical dilemmas, social dos and don'ts, and was capped with Abby's own strongly worded resolution that might be anything from compassionate wisdom to snarky rebuttal.

Everyone was entertaining. There was no one I knew who had the paper delivered to their home and didn't read Dear Abby. I ate up every glimpse I had into the disruptive, unsettled lives of strangers, thrilled to have a peek into an adult's shattered life. It was fun until the day I came across this letter, the essence of which I reconstruct as memory.

Dear Abby,

I am engaged to a wonderful woman. Throughout our relationship we've been open about past relationships, but there is one thing I've been keeping from her. You see, about fifteen years ago, when I was twelve years old, I was sexually molested by my uncle. I spent a lot of time with my uncle

before any of this happened. He was a favourite amongst all the nephews and nieces, but he
seemed to prefer my company above everyone
else's. I didn't have a lot of friends so the extra
attention he gave me made me feel special. I'm not
sure how and when the physical part started — it
happened so gradually and slowly. I never liked the
physical stuff, but I did like my uncle and didn't
want to lose his friendship. He told me never to
tell anyone, that they wouldn't understand, so I
kept it a secret. We continued like this for months
until one day my mom and dad come home and
caught us. I don't remember much of what happened afterwards, only the shocked and horrified
look on my parents' faces. The next day my uncle
committed suicide. Not too many people knew
about this. I am too ashamed and embarrassed to
talk about it. I want to go into this marriage with
no secrets, but I'm terrified that she'll reject me
should she know about such a lurid past.

Signed,
Shameful Secret Past

I had found an unexpected release from all doubts that held me
to a belief that what my dad and I did was just harmless, inappropriate guy behaviour. But there was more in the letter to Dear Abby
than simple validation of my fear and shame. I had been given a
glimpse into the future. This letter to Dear Abby was evidence of
survival, but evidence, too, that guilt, shame, humiliation, and fear
would also survive. How terrifying it must have been for the writer
(if he were at all like me, and I imagined him to be exactly like me),

who at twelve years old experienced the one horror he was most terrified of ever having to face; to have heard the door open and know that there would not be enough time to find a way to fake normal. He must have felt as if death itself was coming through the door.

"I don't remember much of what happened afterwards," the letter stated, "only the shocked and horrified look on my parents' faces." The writer, then a man, but once a boy, appeared in my thoughts as he did at twelve years old, exactly how I imagined myself to look: pale, skinny, dark hair, a stretch of bone and flesh lying across the bed naked and vulnerable. Details of the boy's face were vague, but what need did I have for written descriptions when I understood fully, instinctively, the knotted contortion of grief and destruction etched into his face — an image I feared and imagined as part of a new routine. And neither did I require much in the way of description to understand the crushing numbness of shock in the faces of the parents who open a door a witness their son's degradation. My imagination refused to go further than the door opening. It was enough for me to know that getting caught was not just a possibility, but likely.

And when that happens — then what?

As always, Dear Abby had a response, again, reconstructed here being faithful to the letter's essence more so than how it originally appeared.

Dear Secret Past,

Let me be frank — you have done nothing shameful. This letter is not "your confession." The guilty person is not you. The guilty person was your uncle. I gather that since you have moved on with your life and have formed a relationship, that you received the counselling and care you needed. Your question is whether you should tell your fiancée, and to deal with that aspect of your letter I respond: Yes, tell her. She deserves to know — not because this is a blemish on you, but to allow her the opportunity to be supportive, and to understand her husband. This will also open the door for her to feel comfortable sharing anything in her past she might have been holding back. Yes, there is a risk that her response might be negative, but it's a risk that needs to be taken. Please tell your fiancée. If you were meant to be together, this will bring you closer. But you are asking for much more in your letter than permission to tell your fiancée about a difficult moment in your past. You are asking for permission to be forgiven for a crime that was never yours. You were the victim. Your uncle's decision to take his own life has added to your guilt. It is not the child's responsibility to monitor the deeds and misdeeds of his caregivers. Such an abominable disruption of a child's growth at the hands of an adult is deplorable, selfish, criminal behaviour, but never is it the child's crime. This is not your crime.

These childhood traumas have repercussions that can stay dormant for years until later in life, coming out in unexpected, and sometimes destructive, ways.

It may be that you have already put in the work that is needed, in which case, I applaud your parents and others, including yourself for getting you the help that's needed. Seek out whatever counsel you find the most rewarding, whether it's medical, psychological, or spiritual. There are many organizations and institutes in place where you can go to.

Signed,
Dear Abby

Dad was in the garage. He had the lawnmower blade gripped firmly in a vice that's mounted to the wooden workbench. Dad was running a metal file against the blade's edge using quick, short strokes. The sound of metal scraping against metal is surprisingly smooth and pleasing, sending off a crisp "ring" that resonates with a deep chime. He noticed me but kept working. I tried not to get too close in case it was misinterpreted as an invitation.

"Dad?" I tried to steady the quiver in my voice. Dad despised weakness.

"Hm. Hmm?" He was in a good mood.

"I read something in the paper," I said.

He looked down, smiled at me. It was almost fatherly. A parent reassuring his child that his worst fears were unfounded.

"You read the Dear Abby letter, didn't you?"

So, he saw it, too. He put the file down on top of the wooden workbench. I thought he was going to put his hands on my shoulders, comfort me, and tell me that everything was going to be fine. That he now understood how much what he had been doing was hurting me. He would tell me that it wouldn't happen again and that from now on he was going to be a real father to me.

"Don't worry," he said, "I would never do anything that crazy."

Crazy? Like what? Because the list of crazy things he wouldn't do is pretty short.

"Hush," I said, but I could tell the Wild Boy was in no mood to be quiet.

Good Lord. You know what he's thinking, don't you? He thinks you're worried he'll commit suicide.

No. That can't be. Could he have really thought I was worried about him committing suicide?

I almost missed that part in the letter where the uncle took his own life. What I hadn't missed was Dear Abby's response. Maybe Dad didn't read down that far. I was thinking about the problems that might arise years later: the unspeakable crime, the "abominable disruption of a child's growth at the hands of an adult," the "deplorable, selfish behaviour," the "repercussions that can stay dormant for years until later in life, coming out in unexpected, and sometimes destructive ways," and this mysterious thing Dear Abby called "trauma." But the Wild Boy wouldn't let me finish my thought. He was certain about one thing, and one thing only.

The garage became a vacuous cavern, the tools, the workbench, even my dad, faded into the walls until they were nothing but a rock wall of ruts and jagged edges.

No, you weren't. Of course, you weren't. Who could possibly read that letter and make it about the uncle? Oh, wait a second — you know who might do that? Your dad. Right? After all, isn't that why the guy wrote in to Dear Abby? Was it because of the difficulties he was having dealing with the untimely death of his dear, caring uncle? Yeah, no. I don't think so, either. But that's the way your dad thinks. Sorry to say, but he's not wasting time worrying about you. The Wild Boy stopped, as though he was sincere about being sorry. He looked at me like he was watching for signs of a reaction. As if he had gone too far and was now waiting for the fallout. I could be wrong, but in the pause between his expectation of a reaction, and the realization that I had none to give, I thought I noticed disappointment in the Wild Boy's eyes. *So, now you know. My best guess is that you learn to accept it.*

But I didn't know what it was the Wild Boy wanted me to accept. It annoyed him, I think, for me to not be on the same thought path as him, but he was often far too radical for me to keep up with. If it wasn't one injustice against me that he was railing against, it was another. Most often, though, it was against my dad. That much I understood.

It's what you've been thinking all along, the Wild Boy said, *But I get it. It's not a nice thing to admit to. Even a worse thing, I guess, to know it's true.*

What? I wondered. I still had no idea what the Wild Boy was going on about. But he just smiled at my ignorance, almost as if he was enjoying it. No, not almost. The Wild Boy *was* enjoying this.

You've been thinking that life would be better if your dad were dead, said the Wild Boy.

Jesus Christ — was that true? Is that what I was thinking?

Chapter 11

Most everyone along this stretch of Highway 7 and 8 and up Trafalgar Road and into Waldau Crescent were on their front lawns or in their backyards staring up at the sky as if the moon had suddenly, for the first time, appeared. Radios were on full volume, filling the evening air with the crisp authoritative voices of newscasters giving moment-by-moment accounts as the astronauts prepared to lift off from the moon's surface and begin a long journey home.

Neil Armstrong had set foot on the moon.

"You're witnessing history," said Dad, who I'd never known to show much interest in history before. Who cares about history when all I'm waiting for is a space alien? What good is a moon landing if its only purpose is to debunk fifty years of science fiction movie plots?

Mom flipped her hand and said, "Big whoop. Imagine travelling all that way just to turn around and come back. No siree Bob, you can have it."

Neil Armstrong, who had just set foot on the moon's surface, was back inside the Apollo 11 module with Buzz Aldrin, doing whatever prep work was needed to take off again and reunite with Michael Collins in orbit, having had their brief stopover on the moon before heading back. Doug thought that because he had the same last name as Michael Collins they might be related. I doubted that having the same last name necessarily meant you're related, but Doug had a better chance at being related to an astronaut than I did of being the illegitimate son of James Bond.

"It's the moon. What's the matter with you?" Dad said in feigned exasperation at Mom's dismissal of what was likely this decade's greatest achievement. "Did you think we'd ever see the day when we'd have men land on the moon?"

"I never cared if we did," Mom replied, using a silly cartoony voice that involved enunciating each word an octave higher than the word before. Betty and Fred Chapman laughed.

NASA achieved something far more remarkable I think, than just sending men to the moon; they managed to get Dad to set up extra lawn chairs and invite over the neighbours. Fred, Betty, and Carol were there. Doug, too, of course. Doug and I tried to see if we could spot the Apollo 11 module taking off from the surface of the moon, but even with Mom's high-powered industrial binoculars, we saw nothing but an amplified view of what we could see without binoculars. Carol said she could see it, for sure, sitting there on the moon like a flag-pin stuck into a wall map, and she got so excited by her sighting that I thought maybe she did see something.

"There! There!" Carol bounced with excitement, the binoculars hanging heavy in one hand, her free hand pointing toward the very spot where she's certain the lunar module stands, or perhaps what she saw was the American flag planted and left behind so that eternity, and any future intergalactic explorer, will not forget which nation got there first.

"Mommy, I see it." Carol rushed over to her mother with binoculars in hand.

"Wow," said Betty. "Good for you." Carol dropped the binoculars onto her mother's lap. Betty caught them before they could slip off and fall to the ground. Betty told Carol to be careful, then held the lenses up to her eyes, following the direction pointed out by her young daughter and, yep, sure enough she saw it, too. Or so she said.

The binoculars were now in Dad's hands, and he made a big deal of seeing the rocket.

"Wow, do you ever have great eyes to be able to see that all the way from here." Carol was a favourite of Dad's, and she had come to learn, I think, to anticipate his attention and fawning. Always happy to give her pushes on the swing, rides in the wheelbarrow, and do just about anything to make her laugh. Doug had another look and — he's not sure, but maybe — wait a second — yep, right there — maybe the spaceship or maybe it's the flag — couldn't tell which. I didn't know how anyone could tell with only a quarter of the moon showing and every dark speck on its surface resembling everything and yet nothing. It was my turn to have another look.

"Oh yeah, I see it now," I said, because maybe I did see something and maybe I didn't. What was abundantly clear was how dreary a moon landing could be without aliens. I wasn't the only one whose interest was waning: Carol moved from Betty to Fred to Mom and then Dad, holding the top of a dandelion beneath their chins to see if she could spot a yellow reflection that determined whether they liked butter, and Doug had turned his attention to a renegade grasshopper that continued to elude his capture. Even the adults sitting in their lawn chairs holding their drinks switched their conversation from moon landings to lawn care (no doubt initiated by Carol's dandelion-butter survey) and family summer vacation spots and the kind of things that made grown-ups laugh at their own jokes. There was danger in this sudden dip in enthusiasm for the moon landing that threatened my late night freedom, but

I was too slow to prevent it from happening. I was unable to come up with a suitable way to bring things alive again — to give back to this moment of history a level of credence that would distract Mom from noticing that I was still up and out and playing. Whatever there was about this night that was special enough to bend the rules had run its course.

"Okay, you." My heart sunk. The jig, as they say, was up. "Let's go. It's past eleven. Time you were in bed."

Why did it always have to be my mom who broke up the party and, worse, why did she insist on announcing to the entire neighbourhood that I must go to bed? You never heard Doug's parents calling him in or even Carol's, and I'm older than Carol. I would protest, but since I had already beaten the system by about two hours, I conceded defeat without much more than a disgruntled whine.

"Eleven p.m. already?" said Betty, "Come on Carol, time we got you into bed, too." Carol's protest had a bit more oomph behind it than mine did, but I'd already folded, so there was little hope of Carol getting a reprieve, at least not with my mother setting parental standards for the entire neighbourhood. Doug didn't care. He wanted to go home, anyway, because there was a good movie on late — *The Creeping Terror*. Why couldn't Mom have said that? Why couldn't she have yelled, "It's well past eleven, Thom. Time to come in and watch *The Creeping Terror*"?

The moon could not be seen from my bedroom, but by staring through the open window into an endless dark sky, I could imagine it, shining like it were the only lit ornament on the Christmas tree. I imagined how the moon must have appeared to the astronauts when they broke through whatever wall separates sky from space, to suddenly be hurled into the centre of a vast and dark eternity. And then, to land, to feel first contact with the soil of an untouched planet beneath the weight of the capsule. Then, to prepare themselves, physically and psychologically, for the moment they opened the door, revealing what billions of people have speculated about for centuries. And then Armstrong lowering himself out of the capsule so he could make "one small step for man, one giant leap for mankind."

I closed my eyes and concentrated until I was one with Neil Armstrong. I did this well enough to be able to feel and sense what I imagined Armstrong had felt and sensed. And not just with Armstrong. I did this with anyone, or anything: a person, a pet, a fly, an ant. I would lie in bed and concentrate very hard. There's a name for this: *transcendental meditation*, and I first heard about it from Dennis. But just because I heard about transcendental meditation from Dennis doesn't mean I learned it from him. That skill I would develop years later from watching *The Other*. There's a kid in that movie who's my age. His grandmother teaches him how to enter the spirit of an eagle, and for a time the boy becomes the eagle, feeling the sensation of the wind that kept him aloft, looking down to see not just farm and home but his grandmother and even his own image standing in the field with his eyes closed. I did the same thing the grandmother told the boy to do, to close the eyes, concentrate, imagine, and practise. It worked.

Dennis had a book that talked all about transcendental meditation. Dennis said that when you become good at transcendental meditation, you could project your image to other places so that when you imagine walking over to a friend's house, your friend could see you even though you might still be lying in your bed at home with your eyes closed. Doug and I tried to visit each other using TM but it didn't work. Doug said it was because we were doing it at the same time so while my image was at his place, his image was at mine, and so we kept missing each other. If it could work, I'd have transcendentally meditated myself over to his place to watch *The Creeping Terror*.

I woke the next morning in a world where men had conquered the moon, and already the news seemed old. What didn't seem old, and what I didn't forget, was that Doug had gone home to watch *The Creeping Terror*. First thing on the agenda was to drag every gory, frightening, horrifying *Creeping Terror* detail out of Doug. Hearing Doug retell the plot of a horror movie was almost better than the movie. His retelling of *Lord of the Flies* was filled with beheadings, violence, and graphic torture, so much so, that when I finally saw the movie, I couldn't help being disappointed.

I had slept in. I heard Mom leave through the back door. She muttered something about filling the car up with gas before coming back.

Dad said, "No rush, I got plenty to do around here," and closed the door behind her. I looked at my clock. Nine a.m. The equivalent of noon in our family. Was it too late for me to go with her? What if I jumped out of bed, got dressed, and hopped inside the Rambler before the garage door was even open? But what if she said no? What if she said, you stay here with your dad? I'd be left there, standing with no place to go. Was she just filling the car with gas, or would she be gone longer? Not that it mattered; five minutes or five hours, Dad didn't need a lot of time. I stayed in bed, pretended to be asleep. Maybe he'd leave me alone. Maybe he had something better to do. Surely there were leaves that needed raking.

The garage door opened, and soon after the Rambler's engine kicked in. I listened as Mom backed out of the garage, a distinct shift in sound as the wheels transfer from the garage floor and onto the asphalt. Dad moved from the back door toward the front of the house; Clancy followed. I imagined Dad standing at the front window waving goodbye as Mom turned the Rambler onto the highway, the engine picking up speed until the car could no longer be seen or heard. Dad watched a bit longer, making certain she had gone. A few more seconds of silence before he told Clancy to "stay" and "lie still." With Clancy settled, he moved toward the bottom of the stairs. I prayed that he would continue walking, out the back door, through the breezeway, and into the yard. But I knew better than to think God had time to answer my prayers. Dad started up the stairs. His steps were slow and deliberate as if to not wake me. My own terror was creeping up on me. I turned away from the door and closed my eyes. He reached the top of the stairs. I felt the shape of his shadow in my doorway, clouding whatever light came from the hall; I felt the weight of his presence hovering over me. His eyes alert for any sign of movement. I held my breath, willed myself to be invisible, hidden beneath a heap of bedsheets and blankets.

"I know you're not asleep." He didn't wait for a response but crawled under the blankets beside me. He pressed up behind me. Of course, he knew I wasn't asleep.

"Where's Mom?"

"Oh, don't worry about her," he said his hand reached around my torso, pulling me in tighter. "We got plenty of time."

His fingertips grazed my stomach, fiddling an inch below my navel.

"You got nothing to worry about," he said as he slowly lifted the waistband of my pyjamas.

I didn't even know the Wild Boy was in the room until I heard him speak. Had he been there all night? For him I opened my eyes — what did it matter now, anyway? Dad had already made it known that a sleeping Thom was not necessarily a safe Thom.

Hear that? You got nothing to worry about, right?

It was almost amusing how cavalier the Wild Boy was. Had Dad's routine become so common that even the Wild Boy accepted it as just the way things were? *Tell you what, you finish up here with your "chores," then meet me outside. We'll go down to the bridge and wait for the trains to pass. What do you say?*

What did he expect me to say? *Sounds good. I'll finish up here and be right out.* Was this all becoming so natural that even I was now expected to take this in stride?

Chapter 12

So, *what's it like? I'm not judging, I'm just curious.*

The Wild Boy knew he had no right asking such questions. He had no right to talk about it at all. Prying. I tried to ignore him, but he stayed, sitting there like he was waiting for a movie to start. All he needed was the popcorn.

All I'm saying, is from what I see — it doesn't look like fun. It looks weird, like some kinda disproportionate wrestling match. One that you always lose.

What the Wild Boy didn't understand — what he never understood — was that I had a home. I had the freedom of living outside the city. I had acres and acres to play in. I was one of the lucky ones.

Right. Not every kid is lucky enough to be adopted. The Wild Boy had a phenomenal ability to gauge what I was thinking. It was futile, sometimes, to try to keep my thoughts to myself.

Sometimes I thought that he thought he was being funny when he wasn't. I knew I was lucky to have a family and parents who housed and fed me.

Uh-huh, and who threatened you.

Parents who took me on vacations, I told him.

And snuck into your room at night.

Parents who bought me clothes.

Just to take them off you.

Parents who celebrated my birthday.

But would have preferred you to stay young.

Parents who made sure I had a Christmas tree, who left me presents. Parents who gave me an allowance, took me to movies, did my laundry, cooked my meals, bought my favourite cereal ...

... molested you on a regular basis. But, just a side note, since when has Shredded Wheat been your favourite cereal?

Out of all the little boys my parents might have chosen, they chose me. And how would the Wild Boy have me thank them? By whining and complaining because "Daddy has a little game he likes to play"? Boo-hoo-hoo! I refused to be seen as an ingrate. I refused to overreact or be petty.

Plus, in the end you only have yourself to blame.

Plus, in the end I only have myself to — what?

What?

You said I only have myself to blame.

Doesn't sound like something I'd say.

But you did.

So, I did, and what of it? It's not something you haven't already thought yourself. So much easier to blame yourself than those responsible.

Like who? Dad? I blame him plenty.

How about your mother? Where was she?

The Wild Boy had a lot of atrocious notions and ideas, but to blame my mother? I couldn't let him blame Mom. But it was too late. The Wild Boy was off and running.

For some reason, your mom's off-limits. Funny how she's right on top of things when you sneak off to play in Montag's barn after she told you not to, or grab an extra cookie out of the jar, or waste your allowance on foolish things like movies and comic books. Able to nip all the big issues in the bud before you start listening to rock music, staying out all night, smoking cigarettes, and subscribing to National Lampoon *magazine. The small, insignificant things like being molested daily by your father over the past several years — that's something that can so easily get missed in the daily grind of parenting. Can't really expect her to catch everything, can you? Not even that time Mom came home early …*

Oh, Christ. How I hated when he would bring up that day.

Dad and I on the living room couch. He had a handheld back massager that would vibrate. I was terrified of being electrocuted. It was the middle of the day, and I had warned Dad that Mom could walk in at any moment. He said not to worry, that we would hear her when she drove in (the responsibility for us not being discovered was never his alone). But she did drive in and neither of us heard her, and as soon as the back door opened (small miracle because she could have just as easily come through the front), I jumped up yelling, "I told you, I told you she'd be home."

And Mom slipped into her comedy routine.

"What? What? What did I miss?' she said as if she walked in on a family-fun event.

Oh, Lord, but your dad's face was something furious like he was ready to murder you on the spot. But you're a quick thinker and said, "Dad was tickling me and wouldn't stop ha ha ha." Your mom bought it, or at least gave the impression of buying it. You know what I think? I think you oughta start small. When you can't talk to the majors, you speak to the minors. Tell Doug. Consider it practice. See what kind of reaction you get. Tell him like you're telling him a dirty joke. Tell Doug. Just blurt out, "Hey, guess what, Doug? My dad forces me to have sex with him." It would be like shoving his head into a bucket of ice water. See what happens. It couldn't hurt.

But it could hurt. What the Wild Boy didn't get was that he had nothing to lose. I risked losing everything.

The Wild Boy had hopped onto a new train of thought. He'd do that, present an idea without a follow-through — of course, that's exactly what he'd have said of me. If we had managed to come together on an idea or two, we might have achieved something. The Wild Boy was full of ideas and solutions, all of them radical, careless, and extreme. Me? I was cautious, uncertain, and thought about the consequences.

What about that day you and Doug were back in Montag's woods? What was it he asked? What's up with your dad? Kind of a weird question when you think about it. Makes you wonder if Doug's got a secret to keep, too. If you ask me [which I hadn't], *your dad's running a well-oiled machine — one that moves along quite nicely without creating much noise. No noise, in fact. Wouldn't be so surprising if maybe ... well ... if maybe you aren't the only one.*

Of course, it was ludicrous for the Wild Boy to suggest what he was suggesting. The thing going on between Dad and I was just between Dad and I. Period. It stayed between us. To believe that there could have been others would have meant something else about Dad altogether. It would have meant that he'd been down this road before, that his coy play of innocence (that this was all new and strange to him, too) was a well-rehearsed performance, and the words he used to reel me in and earn my silence were to a well-tested and effective formula. The Wild Boy was wrong about there being others, but he might have been right to suggest I tell Doug. A peer. A friend. Why not?

I went to fetch Doug at his home. I used their back door. The front door was reserved for family, salesmen, and special visitors. Back doors were for neighbourhood kids. Doug was finishing up dinner. I could wait for him, which I often did, but this time I suggested he come over when he was done. He said sure, and about twenty minutes later, Doug shows up in my backyard.

Doug and I had reached an age when real conversations about real topics — women's rights, racial equality, religion — were just us test driving the opinions handed down to us from television shows. I was about to introduce a subject that could have potentially put us on a whole new level of conversation. I really needed to think things out, plan, and rehearse what I was about to say, but I was lousy at doing any of those three things. And so, as ill-equipped as I was at dealing with confessions and admissions, I allowed myself to just say it: "My dad makes me do stuff with him," I said.

I assumed that we both knew what *stuff* meant.

It was the wrong approach. I knew that immediately. Not because of the shocked look on Doug's face, but because of the way the words felt when leaving my mouth. I didn't experience relief, no weight off the shoulders. I felt only regret. I had to take it back. I had to reverse the words. I had to swallow everything I said even though I said very little. I had to rein the words back in before they drifted too far.

"Just kidding," I laughed, but even if it were a joke, it was a horrifying and ugly joke that couldn't be easily dismissed.

It was impossible to gauge whether Doug believed me or not: believed that it was true or believed I was kidding. He had two options to choose from.

"I'm kidding. I'm kidding," I said, but Doug wasn't laughing. His face transitioned from fresh-faced, healthy country boy to sickly, pale kid. He looked at me as if recognizing, for the first time, an insanity that he hadn't noticed before. No amount of laughing or attempting to reassure him that it was all a joke could save me. Doug said he didn't feel well and that he needed to go home.

The Wild Boy was pretty sure that Doug was about to throw up.

"But I'm kidding," I repeated. "You know that, right?" I said, pleading, fearing the worst. Fearing that the Wild Boy had duped me into confessing something I never wanted to confess. Worse, that finally someone had heard me.

"Yeah. I know," Doug said, but he went home, anyway, walking the distance between my house and his with his head down, a kid with too much knowledge.

I spent the rest of the day waiting for the phone to ring. For Rick, Doug's older brother, to come knocking on the door. I waited for my world to come crashing around me. I would've denied it, of course. I would've made out Doug to be a liar, no question. No one called. No one came to the door. So, either Doug kept quiet, or no one was willing to believe him. After all, you don't just go around making accusations against your neighbour based on the unsubstantiated blurting from a problematic preteen.

Still, the Wild Boy hounded me to talk, in ways that were too vague to hold on to. Nothing I could point to and say, "Stop saying that." Even so, I tried to appease his impatience. I told the Wild Boy of my plan to start praying and turn things over to God.

God? You're turning this problem to God, are you? Going right to the top?

I should have known the Wild Boy would have seen this as a foolish resolve. There are few things the Wild Boy mistrusts more than prayer and religion.

Thom. This is God. Got your message. Really? This is not something you can deal with yourself. For Christ's sake, handle this. He's your father. Honour and obey. It's as simple as that. I couldn't have made it any clearer. Look, I gave my son up to be crucified and did he complain? No. Well, once, but that's it. But with you it's over and over and repeatedly; Dear God this and Dear God that ... It gets old. What would you rather? Would you rather your dad nails you to a cross? It could be arranged, you know. If your father sins, so be it, it's his sin. But if you disobey your father, that's your sin. And don't think I don't know about your excessive masturbating. That's right — hiding under the covers in the dark — we can see you, you know. And we know that you sometimes masturbate thinking about him — what's that all about? And by the way leave Laurel Mitchell out of this. She's far too good for you. Now say Amen and leave me alone until you come up with some workable solutions on your own. I can't hold your hand your entire life. I help those who help themselves.

I allowed for the Wild Boy's sacrilegious parody to run dry. I told him what he did was a sin against God. He said God, if there was a God, was unlikely to spot his little sin hiding behind all the big sins going on around here.

It hadn't occurred to me before that moment that perhaps God wasn't helping because maybe God didn't exist. To think that way was a grave sin, more sinful than anything Dad and I were involved in. And yet, there it was. A thought I could not ignore. A possibility I had to consider.

* * *

Dad was done with me and was busy covering up any evidence that might give away our secret. I thought about the Wild Boy's ridiculous scenario that Dad could be harbouring similar relationships with others, as he was harbouring with me. We had ruled out Doug, but what about other family members? What about the past?

What about my sisters?

And so, I asked. The question just came out of me with no thought of being cautious, no thought of the consequences. Dad reacted as though I had leapt at him from a dark corner. As improbable as it seems, I believed I might have hurt his feelings. How could I — his own son — suggest him capable of such a heinous act?

"Why would you say that?" he asked. "Of course not. I'm their father."

"Oh," I said.

I'm confused. Is he not your father, too? Then … why do you do it?

"Then why do we do it?" I asked.

He's stumped. Was this the penny that needed to drop? Had his eyes been pried open so that only now was he aware of what he's been doing, like a sleepwalker who suddenly wakes and finds himself miles from home? But it wasn't an epiphany that had left him bewildered, but that anyone should ask such a despicable, ugly question.

"It's not the same," he said.

Of course. It's not the same. They're blood; I'm adopted. They're his daughters; I'm barely a son. No, he did not do this to the girls, and what kind of kid wouldn't believe his own adopted father. He had ethics. He would never hurt his girls. I know, because, if nothing else, Dad would not lie. Was he capable of such an atrocity? His look of disgust forced me to turn away. Ashamed to have had such evil thoughts and yet relieved to know that Valerie and Anna were safe. Dad was not altogether a monster.

Chapter 13

My Tom Sawyer routine was rusty. Sawyer could get out of the house before Aunt Polly knew he was gone. But Sawyer's Aunt Polly had nothing on my mom. I didn't even make it to the door.

"And where do you think you're going?" she said, as if it were a question she wanted answered. I knew exactly what she was getting at — the evidence was stacked neatly in my room: piles of two-by-fours, three-by-fours, and sheets of chipboard. I had slept the night before with the smell of cut pine. Not so bad, really.

"Out." I tried to keep my momentum, but my feet grew too big to not stumble and my hands too small to get a proper grip on the doorknob.

"Hold your horses," she said.

Fuck.

"You're going to help your dad with that closet today." Mom's had it in her head that the problem between Dad and me could be fixed by putting us to work on a project. We were to build a closet in my room.

Thom Ernst

"I don't know anything about building closets."

"You'll learn," she said.

From who? Dad? Not fucking likely.

I had long put to rest any expectation of Dad being capable of anything remotely fatherly like teaching his son how to build a birdhouse or a go-kart or a tree fort or a closet. Besides, I already had a closet. Granted, it became less of a place to hang clothes and more of a place to shelve old board games: *Mouse Trap*, now missing the plastic boot that kicks the bucket; *Trouble*, with the little plastic dome gone; and a chess set that hadn't been touched since the day Dad tossed it across the room, infuriated because there were too many stupid rules that no one could understand. (Yes, I am to blame for the intricate details of chess.)

There were other things hidden in this closet: a hoard of Lego pieces and dozens of Hot Wheels with Hot Wheel accessories — all amounting to the things I once cherished but had quietly put aside. Not even a Hot Wheels Criss Cross Crash track set with Power Booster held much interest anymore.

Recently, large boxes, none of which were remotely connected to me, had begun taking over my closet. Sealed in these boxes, along with the stale odour of age and confinement, were things too precious to be stored in a dank basement or stacked in the garage to freeze and soak up gas fumes, and yet not useful enough to be unpacked. My existing closet was a purgatory for scraps of material, old sewing patterns, knitting magazines, a broken pocket watch, and fountain pens.

One box was full of material and sewing supplies that Mom had no use for but couldn't see the sense in throwing away. Another box was packed with knick-knacks, including a white-cushioned wooden music box with a silky red lining that played "Heart of My Heart" when you turned the key tucked in the recess at the bottom; it might have once held jewellery. Packed alongside it were two ashtrays, remnants from Dad's smoking days, one shaped like an overturned miniature black plastic pill hat with the fading and ash-burned image of a smiling young woman, her hair billowing out from an air force issued pilot's cap, wearing a mostly unbuttoned cropped shirt tied at the hem into a bow below her breasts, midriff showing, and skin-tight shorts. The other ashtray was an argyle-patterned bean bag topped with a thin metal plate holding four grooves just the right shape and size to balance cigarettes on. Dig deeper in the box and you'd find Dad's army medals, which he explained away as being merely service awards for his time stationed in London, England, in the days immediately following the Second World War. (Dad doesn't have war stories filled with gore and violence like Uncle Bob. Dad was a peacekeeper.)

"Why would anyone boast about shooting off the top of the head of another man?" Dad would say whenever I asked if he had any gory stories like Uncle Bob's. No, Dad didn't care much for violence. The war stories he shared with me were about the hookers he met up with and how careful you had to be, not because of diseases, but because some of them were Nazi sympathizers who hid razor blades in their pussies.

There was a third box, stacked with photograph journals and at least a hundred loose pictures that never made their way into the pages of a photo album; pictures of my family's life before I come along. For me, these pictures were without meaning, although I'm told they were images of Oma and Opa, my great-uncles and great-aunts. All strangers who scowled at the camera as if they were staring into the sun, each standing stiff and uncomfortable against a backdrop of homes and landscapes that seemed desolate and in need of repair. Most of the pictures were black-and-white and framed with a white glossy border that placed the snapshots further back in a time and era so impossibly ancient that I couldn't imagine them being anything other than a vague reflection of someone's memory. I stared long and hard at each image, trying to merge their past with my present, but they only served as reminders of an unshared history when my sisters were children and my parents were young. It was this box that I found most interesting. I suppressed the urge to set up a Hot Wheels Criss Cross Crash set for one last run, but the box of pictures was too distracting. Dad came up with his toolbox in one hand and a power saw in the other. He found me in my room with the photos dumped out of the box and onto a pile on my bed.

"You're just supposed to move the boxes," he said, "not root through them."

I held up a photo of two little boys who looked like Buster Brown, the animated Dutch boy with the blond bowl haircut and the sharp blue sailor's jacket and shorts who, along with Tige, his dog with the signature black spot over one eye, was the trademark of a popular shoe company. Both boys in the photo looked miserable. Their scowls were beyond the scowls of someone staring into the sun. Their scowls came out of frustration and anger. These were boys who did not want their picture taken.

"Who are they?" I asked.

Dad put down the toolbox and power saw by the stack of two-by-fours, three-by-fours, and chipboard stacked neatly against the far wall to the left of the doorway. He walked toward the bed, which was now pushed to the other side of the room so that one side of the bed pressed against the outside wall by the window.

"Let me see," he said, reaching out his hand. I held the photo out to him. He took the picture from me, and when he looked at it, a slight grimace appeared on his face as if struck by a headache that quickly passed. "Yeah ... You know who that is? Quinnie and me."

I had no idea who was who, though what did it matter since the two boys stood identical in their humiliation and anger. "Our mother dressed us like that."

"How come no one ever smiles in your photos?" I asked.

"What was there to smile about? Kids today have nothing to do but play all day. We had chores. When did we ever have time for fun?" Dad examined the picture closer. "She made us go to school like that. Every day. Long hair. Short pants. The other boys would call us girls and chase us from the boys' side to the girls' side. Dad tried to talk her out of it, but she was determined. Quinnie and I were her youngest, and I guess she wanted to keep us babies for as long as she could. I don't know. She was hoping we'd be girls. She'd have put us in dresses if she thought she could get away with it. Short pants were bad enough. Be grateful you don't have to go through that."

Dad lay on the bed beside me. I waited for it; that thing that always happened when he's on my bed. First there would be a few moments of feigned interest in whatever I was doing, a bit of distracted kindness, and then the shifting of his body as he moved closer to me, the hand sliding onto my knee resting there with only his thumb caressing me — of course none of this was as bad as being sent to school with long hair and short pants, mind you. But this time when his hand reached out, it was not for me but for more photos. For the next forty minutes, we went through the pictures, Dad telling me who everyone was, where they were, what was going on. There was a photo of Dad as a young soldier in uniform, standing in front of a large army tent. Dad said he was in the army, but he was never a soldier. Then there was a picture of Mom and Dad on their wedding day standing in front of what could be a rose bush. Mom was pretty but wore a simple dress. Dad was in a simple suit, dark jacket and white pants. There was no church, or guests, or any indication other than their clothes and their smiles to mark the day as a celebration — not at all like the storybook weddings celebrated by Valerie and Anna.

Then there was this picture: a coffin. The coffin lid was open revealing not just the torso, but the entire length of the woman lying in it. She looked, as was often said of people before they're buried, to be sleeping. She wore wire-rimmed glasses and a wrinkle-free dress that draped down to her ankles. The only remotely extravagant part of the dress was the white lace collar around her neck. Dad and I had been going quietly through the photos without much comment, but I broke the silence to ask about this photo and the woman in it. I held out the photo to Dad.

He looked at the picture and was unable to speak. He didn't even move to take the picture from me.

"That's her. That's my mother," he said, and when he did reach to take the picture from me, he did so with such caution and care that I thought perhaps I had come upon something too sacred and delicate to hold. This was a new kind of silence. It was the silence of someone recalling a great sadness, the silence of someone steeped in an unforgettable loss. Dad had regressed so far into his past that I felt as if I'd been abandoned in the parking lot of a rural gas station, watching the churned-up dust and gravel caused by the wheels of his car as he made a quick getaway. Except I could see him. He was still there, lying on my bed, staring at the picture; but in his mind, he was standing alongside his mother's coffin, saying goodbye to her for the final time, all over again. It was in this moment, while watching my dad disappear in the memory of a lost parent, that I felt something close to empathy. Nothing quite as grand as that, but something that could have arguably been said to be drawing me closer to the edge of caring. I didn't like it. Not at all. In the multitude of corrupt and vulgar ways Dad was willing to expose himself, it was this raw, base love for his dead mother that I found to be the most obscene. Such piety in his grief. Unearned. How is it that a man so careless with his affections could grieve so deeply? And my thoughts drifted to images of him lying in his coffin, his eyes closed, his face powdered and pale, his arms tucked straight alongside him — lying at attention, if such a thing is possible — and me standing there, trying desperately to feel something. Would I, too, experience the pain of loss and regret? I needn't have asked. I knew the answer. No. I would not feel pain or regret. I couldn't. My right to mourn a lost parent had been taken from me. I've been robbed of it twice, once with my birth parents and now him. I gave him his moment. What else was I to do?

* * *

Mom came to check on our progress, but not without bringing us sandwiches, like a ranch wife taking food out to her men working in the field. She brought bottles of soft drinks. It was all very 1950s — a Coca-Cola ad painted by Norman Rockwell. Dad and son working together.

"The closet's not going to build itself," she said.

* * *

Mom had us building a closet so that father and son could build a relationship. She imposed, I think, a wisdom worthy of King Solomon, tackling unconventional problems with unconventional solutions. Mom knew that even at this late stage in the tarnished and unrepairable relationship between the boy and the man, there was a primal urge for a son to have a father. She was determined to see this through, even if the father, in this case, was my dad.

* * *

Dad sighed so deeply and sorrowfully that I was reminded of something Carol once said to me when she was little. She said that a sigh was the sound of an angel escaping the soul.

She couldn't have been more than five at the time. I thought about the angels locked in Dad's soul struggling for their freedom, and I wondered if they might look like the angel Mom saw outside her bedroom window so many years ago. I wondered, too, about the angels in my soul, and if they were to ever find their way out, would they rather strike me down with a flaming sword than allow me to live and further corrupt the world?

"Right," Dad said, moving out of the past and back into the present, tossing the picture of his dead mother back in the box where it was once again buried to be forgotten in a lost pile of memories. "Let's get this thing started."

We moved to the stack of two-by-fours and three-by-fours, the chipboard panels, the tool box, and the power saw. Building a closet; a father and son bonding project when, to my thinking, there was far too much bonding going on already.

I was surprised by how much I liked the idea of carpentry work, of building something, handling a hammer and nail, saw and wood, of watching something rise from nothing to become something. I liked it even more when there was a power saw involved. I wasn't convinced Dad was enough of a handyman to teach me anything about carpentry. I imagined him to be no better at it than me. But then I was hit with the revelation that Dad in fact could spearhead such a project. He knew about building closets. He knew construction things. Things that only good fathers knew, because there is something about working with your hands to build that was chaste and pure and decent, something spiritual and soulful. I related none of these things to Dad. There is an art to building, to using clean white wooden planks, smooth puzzle pieces waiting to be put together to turn an empty space into a usable space. Who knew Dad had this in him? I edged dangerously close to feeling pride watching Dad measure and cut the wood, assembling it so that it made sense. The two-by-fours and the three-by-fours made the frame. The existing walls of my bedroom made up the other sides. Shelves were put in between the sides, and one big shelf on the top. A metal rod stretched the width of the closet space, and a door, remarkably fitted perfectly into the doorframe. This really was going to end up looking like a closet. How did he do it? Where did he find the time or energy to achieve anything beyond the gargantuan effort it took to maintain our secret?

This was Dad's chance to be a father. Dad's chance to teach me about building, about carpentry, and about taking pride in your work. In a few days, there would be a closet where there once wasn't one, if only he could make it through to the end without a break to relieve his urges.

But he couldn't. Any expectation that the ruins of our relationship could be salvaged were dashed. The more walls that went up, the more places there were to hide, and the more opportunities there were for a quick grope. There was nothing so sacred, chaste, and innocent that my dad couldn't turn ugly.

Chapter 14

Clancy had been slowing down for a while, it was hard to not notice. She stopped scrambling for attention the way she once did, she no longer twisted in circles in front of the door, anticipating Dad's coming home; there were no anxious whines and pleads to be let out for a run, or to chase after whatever scent she picked up. She would rest her head on Dad's lap while he scratched behind her ears, rubbed her snout, once a beautiful ginger-red, now turned grey.

"She's getting old, Clare," Mom said. "Poor old thing. Aren't you, girl?" She bent down to pat Clancy gently on her shank. The beast she swore she'd turn into a rug became the recipient of her empathy and care. Dad still took Clancy when he went outside, but the dog simply followed where she once ran circles around him, darting off ahead, turning around, and racing back to his side. Dad would coax her forward with every step. The dog moved cautiously, as if walking on ice, her back legs trailing with the hint of a limp. There was less sheen to her coat, and the fur felt coarse rather than silky. But her greatest love was still with Dad; her tail still wagged when she sensed he was home or when he entered a room. So, Dad would find her a shaded spot to lie under away from the heat of the sun, beneath a tree or the shadow of the house, while he raked leaves, or mowed the lawn, or tended to the rows of raspberry bushes that filled the two acres of land where Clancy once ran.

I'd been avoiding Clancy, though I would not have done it consciously. Even so, my avoidance, was a pure act of selfishness. I didn't — or couldn't — deal with watching her struggle, seeing her stumble when lifting off the ground or bending down to sit, or yelp unexpectedly from pain she was unable to tell us about, to notice the glassy, cold distance in her eyes and wonder why she looked so sad.

Clancy no longer barked at the paper boy or growled when a stranger came to the door. She still wailed when Dad played the bagpipes, but her cry became more severe and her discomfort not as comical as we once could get away with believing, so Dad put the bagpipes away, and without Clancy's accompanying howl, he lost all interest in playing. And then the seizures. We didn't recognize them as seizures at first. They began as mild muscle spasms, stiffening joints that left Clancy unable to stand or to sit up. Clancy's feet slid beneath her, symptoms easily mistaken as a malady of another sort, exhaustion, maybe, old age, for sure, but nothing so serious as a seizure. But by this Sunday there was no mistaking how bad Clancy's health had become.

We were sitting down to dinner with Aunt Rhea and Uncle Gord. Aunt Rhea had called in the morning announcing that they were coming for dinner. If Mom couldn't come up with a reasonable excuse as to why they shouldn't come, they'd be at our door a few hours later. I picked up from conversations that Aunt Rhea and Uncle Gord weren't as smart as the rest of the family. And there was something unusual about Aunt Rhea's face; it was fleshy and squished so that her cheeks and chin and mouth collapsed like someone without dentures, her bottom lip protruded into a pout and was constantly being pushed at with her tongue as if tongue and face were vying for optimal position.

"It's like watching a cow chewing cud," Mom once said.

To which Dad snapped back, "It's not her fault. That's the way she was born." He protected Aunt Rhea.

Aunt Rhea heard it first, a sorrowful cry like wind rushing through a hollow reed, coming from the breezeway where Clancy often stayed on hot days. Aunt Rhea wondered if she hadn't heard a cat or another animal in heat. Dad knew it was Clancy. He left the table without bothering to swallow the food in his mouth. The rest of us followed.

Clancy laid on the cushions Dad set out for her, motionless except for her snout opening and closing, biting the air, and her eyes darting up and down. Dad knelt by his dog and stroked her coat, speaking to her softly, calming her, telling her that everything's okay — but we knew it wasn't. It was the most compassionate thing I'd seen Dad do. And then came a second howl more mournful than the first and far more terrifying. It hadn't come from Clancy; it was coming from Mom. Mom had her eyes covered and her face buried into Aunt Rhea's shoulder. This made me start crying, too. It embarrassed me, crying in front of my uncle and aunt, my dad and mom, but watching our dog die, and hearing Mom cry, was too much for me. Too much for all of us, I think. Freddy Chapman was in his backyard, feeding the chickens. He heard us and came over. He saw Dad leaning over his dog.

Clancy didn't die. She lived but was weak and in pain. Dad knew it was time for Clancy to go. Freddy offered to take Clancy to the vet if it was too much for him. No. Dad thanked Freddy, but he thought it best if he did it.

When I came home from school the next day, Dad was in the backyard working, Mom was sitting in the front room quietly

knitting. Clancy was gone. I didn't see or hear much from Dad
over the next few days. He kept to himself. Missing his old friend,
I guess. Even if we did happen to be alone together, he didn't come
near me. Didn't even acknowledge that I was there. It was strange,
but it was wonderful to be left alone. Weeks went by without incident. I'm sorry Clancy had to die before I felt safe again.

* * *

I was spending the night at Patty and Al's place. Patty and I were
watching *The Tonight Show Starring Johnny Carson* on a night when
Johnny goes into the studio audience looking to see if anyone had
a talent they wanted to share on national television. This guy stood
up and did an amazing Paul Lynde imitation. Patty and I thought
the guy was hilarious, but when Johnny gave the guy a coupon for
a free steak dinner and the guy said, still in a Paul Lynde voice, "I'm
not hungry," Patty and I almost suffocated from laughing. We were
able to calm down enough to breathe again, but then, Patty started
doing her own Paul Lynde imitation, and maybe it wasn't as good
as the guy on the Carson show, but it was just as funny.

We ended up in hysterics again, laughing so hard that I begged
Patty to stop saying "I'm not hungry," no matter how funny it was.
Patty and I were still watching television when Al came home from
work. He was in uniform, and it made me proud to have a cousin
who was a cop. It was great to see Al, but I was afraid that now we'd
have to go to bed, and I wasn't the least bit tired yet. Patty didn't
want to sleep either, and Al said he'd been looking forward for the
chance to sit down, kick up his feet, and enjoy a cold one. It was
strange seeing a cop in uniform slouching on the couch, drinking
a beer; it was like the time I went to Doug's church and afterward
we saw a priest smoking a cigarette. I knew smoking wasn't against
the law, but I was pretty sure it was a sin.

"Sorry to hear about Clancy," Al said. "I know how much Clare loved that dog."

"Yeah."

"Your mom, too, I bet," said Patty. Patty said *I bet* a lot after her sentences — that way she got to ask a question without having to ask one.

"Yeah. I think so. She always complained about Clancy. Used to say she was going to make a rug out of her any time Clancy did something wrong. Never meant it, though. Just something she said."

"Yeah, your mom says some strange things sometimes," said Patty. Then, as if afraid she might have offended me, said, "She's a hoot. Doesn't mean half the things she says. You must've heard it all, I bet."

"Yeah. But ... I don't know ... she's strict. It's more fun here."

"It's always more fun at our house. We're fun people. Aren't we, Al?" But Al was taking a long draw from his beer, looking as if he were capable of staring backward in time, lingering on some nagging bit of police work still clouding his mind. "Al! Isn't that right?"

"Hmm?"

"Aren't we fun people?"

"We're a hoot."

I wish it were Patty and Al who were in Harmony Lunch that day, and it was Al's hand I took and not Dad's. Boys aren't to think such things. Especially adopted boys who are lucky to have a family at all.

Aww, go ahead, think away. Imagine how much better life would be better with Patty and Al. Not only could you go to school and say that your dad was a cop and an OHA hockey star, but you'd be safe with Patty and Al.

"I wish it were you guys who adopted me."

Whoa. Wow. I honestly didn't think you were going to say that aloud. But ... never mind. That's good. That's a good first step. And remember, with Patty and Al, you can tell them anything. Just be sure that when you tell them anything to tell them everything. Someone needs to know. It might as well be a friend.

"Every kid feels that way at one time or another," Al said. "I know I did."

Patty agreed that Mom sure liked to put me down a lot. I hadn't noticed, but it was peculiar that others might think so.

You're on your way. The door's been opened ... relax ... let the words come to you. You got this. You don't even need to work at it. The words are on the tip of your tongue. Just open your mouth and say "aww"... Fuck it, I'm going to talk.

"Christ, my old man used to give me a good smack when I got out of line." Al talked like that, calling his dad "the old man," a disparaging term loaded with affection — too affectionate to comfortably use it when referring to my dad. "Most of the time I deserved it."

Is that right? A good smack? Ah, well, have a seat. Have we got a story for you!

I hated to disappoint, but I was done talking. I understood that the Wild Boy had my interest in mind, but he was dangerously unconcerned of the risks involved. No. Best to keep the secret. Al said that "most of the time he deserved it." Maybe most of the time I deserved it, too.

What? That our name will be mud? Fuck that. Let them call us mud if they want. What's in a name? Sticks and stones.

That's when Al asked if there was anything to eat and suggested we order a pizza. Patty said, in her Paul Lynde voice, "I'm not hungry," which made Patty and me howl, but Al didn't get it and told us that we're both crazy. It was the first time I had pizza. (Pizza was too fancy for my parents. "Who needs it?" Mom would say.) It was the first time I had food delivered to the door. ("If I can't make it myself at home, we don't need it." This would have been Mom again.) And it was the first time I remember staying up this late: 2:00 a.m. Al had the last slice of pizza and finished a second beer. He patted Patty on the knee and said that we should probably call it a night. We all agreed that two in the morning was darn late for a kid my age.

I drifted beneath the wave of hushed voices that came from Patty and Al as they glided through their nighttime routine, a young couple fresh in the stages of a new life together. I slept soundly that night, comforted by the delusion that life would find a way to be this kind forever.

Chapter 15

- - - - - - - - - - -

On a Sunday afternoon in September, I was in the garage standing by the workbench. Mom's car was in the driveway, Dad had left with his car for the afternoon shift at Uniroyal, leaving plenty of room for me to idly drum up ideas for a woodworking project that would end up going nowhere. I had in front of me a collection of wood scraps and an assortment of screws and nails. The screws and nails had been sorted by size and types and placed into baby food jars. The lids had been fastened to the bottom of a mounted two-by-four so that retrieving what was needed meant you only had to twist the jar from the lid. Dad's organizational skills were a thing to marvel at. My weekend visit with Patty and Al inspired me to do something constructive. Building a birdhouse seemed to be the most natural choice. I had no plan. What need did I have for plans? If I were to build a birdhouse, then the birdhouse would look like the tens and hundreds of birdhouses I have seen throughout my life. I was raised on wildlife and nature. If I hadn't already had a clear idea of how a birdhouse should look then I had no right calling myself a country boy.

I was in the imagining stage of designing the birdhouse, deciding how to best utilize the tools and the material I had set out to work with, when Mom came in through the front of the open garage door. Traditionally, if Mom needed me, she'd have shouted from the front doorstep, or, if she was hoping to secure a more personal connection and she knew I was out the back or in the garage, she'd have followed the route from kitchen, down the hallway, out the back door, and through the breezeway.

"What have you been telling people?" Her face hard, her words fired in pronounced, calculated bullets giving her anger an edge of unnerving intensity.

I had been imagining myself as the handy craftsman contemplating the many ways wood can be arranged to take on the shape of a birdhouse, but the moment of being blissfully lost in a daydream was gone. I barely recognized this woman shadowing the frame of the open garage door as my mother; this woman who raged about a grave injustice — a grave injustice that I had committed, to judge from the fierce look in her eyes and in the fury of her voice. It took several beats before registering Mom as "real" and not some twisted hallucination from a daydream gone sour. A few beats more before her words made any sense.

"They said they don't want to spend time with a boy who has no respect for his father," Mom said. She came no farther than the threshold of the garage door. Her anger crushed the warmth and pleasantness from the afternoon. I imagine it would have been impossible for her to resist the impulse to hit me had she been standing closer. Or perhaps my crime was so deplorable to her that to risk standing next to me was to risk staining herself with the residue of my sick, demented sin.

Who is she talking about? The Wild Boy was often a few steps ahead of me, but this time he seemed to be as caught off guard by the attack as I had been. I hadn't any idea who she was talking about. The birdhouse I had built in my mind shattered into splinters and was replaced with a running line of possible people I might have offended. I came up with no one. There were either too few people to consider or too many to remember.

"Who are you talking about?" I asked. The confusion was sincere, and she sensed it. I believed it took her aback. No doubt she was prepared for me to become defensive, to hand her an excuse built upon lies, but I was legitimately baffled. No doubt I was guilty — I just didn't know what it was that I was guilty of.

"You know very well who," she said, as if calling my bluff, although the slight hiccup in her voice suggested that she couldn't be a hundred percent certain that I was bluffing at all. "Patty and Al, that's who."

Patty and Al. My mind traced back to the night before and to every weekend and outing with Patty and Al that I've ever had. What was said? Al, the only older male I knew, besides Wayne, who made it safe to be with an older male, who took me to hockey games, the CNE, stock car races, and baseball games without asking anything in return. And Patty, who talked to me like an adult, and who could make me laugh harder than I did watching a Jerry Lewis movie.

"What did I say?" I'd been blindsided, at a loss as to what sin had been committed.

"You know damn well. You are a disrespectful, disobedient, ungrateful child who doesn't give a damn about this family. I'm sorry we ever took you in, put a roof over your head, food in your stomach, and clothes on your back. I ought to call Children's Aid right now and have them take you back. You make me sick."

The garage, even vacant of its cars and with both of its doors open so that to all appearances it was missing a wall, was too confining to properly shield me from her assault. I was a foreigner who had unknowingly committed an unforgivable affront against local custom and now stood stupidly with hammer in hand, beside a yet-to-be-built birdhouse, waiting for judgment to be passed.

"I didn't say anything." It was true, in so far as I said nothing that I thought would have warranted this kind of anger.

"Bullshit," Mom said. The Wild Boy chuckled at Mom's indiscretion, admiring how much more comfortable and easily the word fell from her mouth than the same type of expression would have come if it were from Dad. "I just got off the phone. I had to listen to all the terrible things you've been saying about your dad. You should be ashamed of yourself."

"Like what? Who called?"

"That's none of your business," Mom said. And then things got weirder. "And what's this about you being glad Clancy died?"

"Clancy." I had to say her name aloud to process from one line of confusing accusations to another. "I never said that. I might have said I was glad she died instead of suffering." It was the only thing that would have made any sense to me at the time. Although, looking back now, I seemed to recall telling someone that I wasn't as upset about Clancy's death as I thought I would be. That, too, could have been because of her suffering. Either way, I was not as callous nor cavalier about losing Clancy as Mom seemed to have been indicating.

"You will not be seeing Patty and Al again," Mom said. "And you better start learning to respect your father." And with that my mother turned her back, leaving me alone, more alone than I might have ever felt before, standing in front of the tool bench, the hammer still in my hands, the unfinished birdhouse that would now stay unfinished.

Mom left, and the bright, sunny day that had motivated me to build with my hands lost its brightness. Lost its brightness not because Mom took the sun with her, but because Mom left behind a bitter darkness. There was nothing more to the day. The day had ended, even though by the standards of time there were still a few hours of daylight left. Without much thought to the process, I put the tiny screws and nails back their baby food jar containers and twisted the jars back onto their lids. I hung the hammer on the hooks against the wall, returned the scraps of wood back to where I had found them. I did all this and then left the garage, though I hardly recall moving at all. I left for someplace outside, someplace where I could work out what it was that went wrong.

Patty and Al. What had happened to make Patty and Al so angry? So angry that they waited until I was gone to huddle together to negotiate my offence so that they — in tandem — could conclude that the only act going forward was to report me to someone, who then reported to my mom.

Patty and Al split up years after they, or someone on their behalf, had called Mom to let us know that Patty and Al had washed their hands of me; that they were done, done, done, done. Al had an affair — I wanted it to be a rumour — and that affair was enough for the golden boy to lose his status as everyone's favourite son. Mom took a firm stand, saying that if you've betrayed one family member then you've betrayed all family members. I was impressed. Apparently, our family had an honour code of which I was totally unaware. We were like gangsters that way.

As to the incident in the garage, there was no discussion or follow-up, no answers, no resolutions. There was just an unspoken agreement to quietly return to the abnormal normality of grappling with life. Mom had mastered a knack of forgetting without forgiving, and I suppose I was expected to take her lead. Life was revealing yet one more level of absurdity for which I wasn't prepared. That I had been selected as the reason that Patty and Al abandoned me was more *adult* than anything I had experienced. Life hadn't stopped as I thought it would. It simply continued leading me along on the same irrational path I've been on since I could remember.

Not such an unusual feeling, I'm sure, regardless of one's life experiences, but a feeling that I believe leaked dramatically into the next day.

Monday. I had hoped to have died by then, avoiding any need to crank out yet another hapless grin. Nothing dramatic, just a quiet death to cover me in my sleep; or, better still, to have vanished, leaving people to wonder if I had ever existed at all. No such luck. The sun rose at seven, the alarm went off at eight, the radio deejays were already cracking up over their own jokes. Life didn't care if I had fallen off the Earth, and it had no intention of slowing down to wait until I was ready to hop back on.

I was a week into Wilmot Junior High, two steps away from childhood and one step toward adolescence. I began the school year alone, having the previous year been randomly selected by Dennis to be shut out from our group of friends. It took the final months of grade six, plus that entire summer, for the wounds from that shock to begin to heal, leaving me scarred forever as an outcast. It was around the time of Dennis's campaign against me that the Wild Boy's visits became more frequent. I didn't mind; in fact, his visits were welcome. It was good timing, as far as I was concerned. He followed me to school, which I hadn't expected. That was new. I never asked, but I suspected the Wild Boy never cared for Dennis or the gang, and that adhering to the group's fickle likes and dislikes, always based on Dennis's whims, took more effort than he thought the friendship was worth. I doubt the Wild Boy cared who befriended him and who didn't. Caring about being liked was my territory. Sometimes I could skip over the "being liked" part, but the "not being liked" part I took very seriously. If a friendship should fall apart or not take off as hoped, I'd fret about it for days, weeks, months. I would make myself sick trying to make amends, to accommodate wherever I could, to do anything to fix it. But the Wild Boy? He'd have moved on before he even knew he wasn't wanted. Wouldn't think twice. The past was the past and that was that. I'm pretty sure he had been hoping for his fuck-you attitude to rub off on me. Guess that's why he stuck around, particularly those first few weeks at Wilmot Junior High. New year, new school, new group of kids. If he could start me off with a solid fuck-you attitude, he'd have placed me well ahead of the game. But I don't know. I was more of a *sure, sorry, whatever you say* kind of guy. I'm pretty sure Dad took the *fuck-you* right out of me.

The Wild Boy stayed close by me that entire Monday, for which I was grateful, after having been ditched, yet again, by another set of friends. Adult friends this time, which tossed me onto a whole new realm of failure. I was now a successful failure on a much higher level.

I shuffled through the day, thinking little, feeling less. This was fine, too. I didn't want to think. Didn't need to feel. I did what had to be done. Even so, even with the Wild Boy marching off on his own without my approval, we were getting through the day with minimal incident. Until Mr. Cressman's history class. That's where things took a turn.

There are many places a twelve-year-old might feel unsafe. A great many of those unsafe places would be at Junior High: the playground, the lunchroom, the gym class, shop class, and on school buses, but not in Mr. Cressman's history class. Cressman could favour an entire classroom and not single out one kid as being better or worse than another.

Cressman was "inclusive" in the way "inclusion" would have been understood by a school of 1970s rural Ontario white kids with yet undetermined sexual preferences. I suspect Mr. Cressman's type of inclusion would work even if he were teaching today, but that's an untested theory, and I've misjudged such things before.

Cressman was thin, possibly scrawny, always wore a suit and tie (invariably a shade of blue, most often navy), had wire-rimmed glasses propped on the bridge of a pointed and slightly bent nose, which poked above a thick black moustache that overpowered a somewhat mousy face. Hardly the winning look of a popular and respected teacher, and yet no one talked back, spoke poorly, or otherwise mistreated Mr. Cressman in any way.

I was in Cressman's class, fourth row, second from the front, when a shift of mood blanketed the room as though a light switch had been flipped off leaving me in the dark. But nothing had changed, as far as I could tell. Until I noticed that something had changed; the Wild Boy had fallen silent and was watching Cressman, scrutinizing him with strained curiosity. I imagined him to be struggling with how it could be that this Sunday school version of Ichabod Crane held such command over a room of twelve-year-olds. Had I not been aware of the Wild Boy's massive lack of concern for classroom rules and etiquette, I might have interpreted his silence as a sudden interest to learn, but the chances of that being true ranged from the unlikely to the impossible. Whatever held the Wild Boy's attention had little to do with a fresh appreciation for the history of Sir John A. Macdonald or William Lyon Mackenzie King. If the Wild Boy's silence was a warning, and I suppose it was, then it was a warning that went ignored.

Cressman courted the class with the facts and rumours of our early prime ministers like he was a man dishing out gossip to a room of meddlers, dazzling us with the eccentric secrets of Mackenzie King, who'd seek advice from his deceased mother and wouldn't move on policy without first consulting his dog. I jotted these points of interest down somewhat absently, and entirely unnecessarily, since these were fun facts and not the intended takeaways Cressman had hoped we'd get from his lesson.

"I don't think you'll need to remember any of this, Thom," Mr. Cressman said, alerted by the rapid tick of my pencil as it struck against the thin divide between my desk and the pages of my notebook. "I can assure you it won't be on any test." The class laughed. It was in good fun — that much I understood, but the best of me could only drum up a hollow smile, which was a weak effort, I felt, in concealing the humiliation of having my invisibility vanish.

Who is this guy? The Wild Boy said. I ignored him. I placed my pencil on the desk to allow Cressman to continue the lesson without the independent pecking sounds of my notetaking.

Cressman thanked me, turned his back to the class and, beneath the name *William Lyon Mackenzie King*, which had already been scrawled across the blackboard, he chalked the words *longest-running P.M.*, *World War Two*, and *Liberal*. I assumed these to be the things about King that Cressman wanted us to remember. I considered writing them down — exactly as they appeared on the blackboard, with *William Lyon Mackenzie King* topping the page and this list of King highlights beneath, but I didn't want to create any further disruption.

"Okay," Cressman said. We had moved well into the afternoon. The countdown toward the end of another school day had all but begun. Cressman's suit jacket was off and hung neatly over the back of his chair. Beneath the jacket he wore a blue-and-white striped shirt, pressed and cleaned, his matching navy-blue tie loosened from a day of wear. "For the rest of the class we're going to read chapter three from our history books. Don't worry. It's a short one. Five pages. And it would be a good time for taking notes — *Thom*." I hadn't expected the emphasis thrown back on me. I can't imagine my smile was any more unconvincing this time than it was the first time around. *Fuck you*, the Wild Boy said beneath his breath. I didn't understand his hostility against Cressman. For reasons only he knew, the Wild Boy had taken an exception to this gentle and wholly approachable man. "The point of this exercise is to see what you can determine from the reading as being important."

Fuck him, said the Wild Boy.

Mr. Cressman stole a look at the clock mounted above the classroom door: 2:45. Thirty minutes before final bell. Textbooks dropped on wooden desktops, sending out popping sounds like bubbles randomly bursting through the room. Pages like paper wind chimes rustled as students rooted through their books in search of the slim-versed chapter three. Notes were being taken and, as was the case with my own note-taking a few moments earlier, an arrhythmic pecking of pencils sounded like irregular-sized raindrops pelting against the notepads. No one's pencil echoed louder, or was more disruptive than mine, and this seemed to heighten the Wild Boy's agitation. As if my frantic scribblings were alerting everyone's attention to us.

The Wild Boy watched Cressman's approach, anticipating the teacher's notice, daring him to utter but one challenging, mocking, hateful word against me. I wished for Cressman to walk by. To skip our row. To be distracted by something, anything. I did all I could to hold the Wild Boy back. Anything to calm him, to not let him get out of control. I tried, but I couldn't.

Let him say something. Just let him say one little thing. The more incensed the Wild Boy got, the harder it was to keep him on this side of silence. Cressman and the Wild Boy were on a collision course that could not be avoided. I struggled to keep focused on my history text, to concentrate and retain some shape of understanding on the tactics and wartime popularity of William Lyon Mackenzie King, but the words I read were meaningless. Still, I refused to lift my head from the text. I struggled to negotiate any comprehension I might glean from the words in front of me. Ignoring Cressman even as he moved closer. Ignoring the Wild Boy even as he grew more volatile.

Cressman strolled along the aisles, down one, up the other, in a manner of leisure rather than authority, peeking over a student's shoulder, checking their work for accuracy and neatness before moving to the next.

There was no chance of my passing the neatness check, considering how frequently I'd been chastised for sloppy penmanship. The greater the effort I put into keeping things legible, the more illegible my notes became. This was the source of my anxiety, and so it became the source of anxiety for the Wild Boy who, I couldn't help thinking, was looking for any excuse that would confirm Cressman as one of the bad guys.

Cressman's stroll eventually led him to hovering over my desk blocking the fragment of light that stood between me and the Wild Boy. Having Cressman loom over me broke the Wild Boy free from whatever thread of control I had tied to him. Then, on a foundation of secrets, shame, fear, and rage, a fire rose and spewed out of him with volcanic force. I've seen people collapsing into epileptic seizures who counted to ten before they lost control of their bodies; I imagined that might have felt like this. The Wild Boy tore into my notebook, ripped at the pages, shredded them as if all that was wrong in my life boiled down to sloppy penmanship.

Mr. Cressman waited for the fury to pass. If the Wild Boy was to be punished for his outburst, he didn't much care. He was beyond that. He simply laid his head on my desk, exhausted and beaten as if his entire being had been filled with hatred, and now that his hatred was spent, he was nothing more than a deflated shell. His breathing became quick and shallow, in and out like a bellows stoking a fire. The teacher's hand fell on the Wild Boy's shoulder, directing him out of the classroom. Cressman spoke softly, calmly, instructed the Wild Boy to take slower breaths. The touch to the shoulder conveyed compassion, a touch without aggression, or intent. I'm unclear as to how the scene played out to the others in the classroom. What did they make out of this storm that blew in from nowhere? An anger unlike any they had known. What were the stories they told at their dinner tables that night? What happened in the classroom when Mr. Cressman guided the Wild Boy into another room?

It occurred to me that Cressman might want to call my home. I begged him not to. I was slowly getting back control, and there was no way I wanted to risk that the Wild Boy's rampage might return.

"My parents aren't home," I told him. "They're busy and they mustn't be disturbed."

Nevertheless, within an hour Mom was at the school office. She didn't seem perturbed by the disruption in her day — I had expected she would be, but neither was there any more concern than if she had come by to take me to a scheduled dentist appointment.

Strange.

There wasn't much exchange between Cressman and Mom. It was as if the worst of everything had come and went — a quick and easy one-size-fits-all breakdown. A single-alarm fire that quickly burned itself out. Still, to be on the safe side, it was suggested that I go to the hospital.

The Wild Boy laid low. I was grateful for that. Mom looked as if she had forgotten about yesterday's garage confrontation. I didn't need her to find something fresh to be angry about.

I sat on the edge of a hospital bed, still dressed, my mother sat on a chair across from me, her purse clutched on her lap. Curtains were pulled around us, offering privacy from the other six beds in the ward. I found hospitals and doctors comforting, I suppose from having often imagined myself as a doctor, but also because of the atmosphere of care. But now I was quiet and intimidated by how foreign it all seemed: the height of the bed, the equipment that hung from the walls, and the doctor, who was Chinese but didn't sound like any of the Chinese people I'd seen in films or on television. For all our talk about equality, race rarely went unnoticed.

The Chinese doctor looked at me. He seemed annoyed. I imagined he had a lot of patients who truly needed his help, and here he was wasting his time on a kid who had a temper tantrum in history class. I wondered what was going on in the other beds nested behind closed curtains. I registered no fever when he took my temperature; my eyes, ears, and throat showed no discernible signs of infections. There was no visible reason for me to be taking up his time.

"What exactly happened?" the doctor asked, no Charlie Chan or Mickey Rooney accent.

"The school said he just started to breathe in and out like he couldn't get any air," my mother answered.

"Has this happened before?" the doctor asked me.

"Nope, never," Mom said.

"Any history of this in the family?" This question was directed at Mom.

"He's adopted. We don't know much about his family history. Only that he was born up near Parry Sound."

The doctor continued to check me, feeling my arms, pressing against the joints and tendons.

And when he was done, "Just open your shirt for me." And I did. I had experience at undressing on command.

The stethoscope pressed on my chest, stomach, and back.

"Everything okay at home?"

The Wild Boy's hand jutted in the air like a student responding to the only question he had an answer to, his voice locked in an octave only I could hear. Well, now that you've asked, Doctor, let me tell you how things are at home. You see — they aren't so good. Dad — we won't call him Father — he hasn't earned that right — has taken up touching Thom in places that, well, I'm certain he's not supposed to be touched. And other things that I'm sure would just embarrass you. Let's just say this: Dad calls them blow jobs. Do you know what those

*are? Do they have blow jobs in China? Dad said he shouldn't tell any-
one, so he's been keeping this a secret for a long time. That's got to mean
Dad knows it's wrong — which is confusing because from the little I
know about being a grown-up, you don't do something you know is
wrong and then teach your children to do the same thing. Dad doesn't
seem to get that even though he goes to church, he goes to work, he
doesn't even swear that much. But I must tell you, Doctor, that these
things he does are not making me like his dad very much.*

*But I really couldn't tell you what's going on because, well, here's
the thing: it's been going on for so long that he feels as if he's just as responsible as Dad is. Dad explained what will happen if anyone finds
out. What did he say exactly? Oh yeah, he said that if anyone finds
out about what they do then their names will be mud. Imagine that.
Mud. That means they will be looked down upon, hated, scowled at,
and chased out of town. Frankly, chase me out of town, I don't give a
damn, but Thom — this kid you're talking to on the bed — he doesn't
want to be chased out of town. So, he's begged his dad to stop, he's
pleaded with him, cried, and tried to appeal to him as a father — but
we've agreed not to call him Father, right? But nothing he's done has
stopped him, Doctor. But that's not the worst. The worst is that, as
much as he hates it, it's become an addiction. Could you help him
with that, Doctor? Could you help him hate it more than he's resigned
to it? Anyway, to answer your question: No, things aren't going well at
home. But whaddya going to do?*

"He and his dad don't get along." It was strange to hear Mom
say this. So, she knows that something's not right. But she was
also saying that not only did I not like my dad, my dad didn't
like me.

"I was asking him," the doctor said sharply. My mother tried to
shrug off the doctor's dismissal, but I could tell her feelings were
hurt. She sat quietly. Obedient in the face of authority.

Too bad you aren't a doctor, the Wild Boy laughed.

But I couldn't talk. I wanted the doctor to know what I knew. I wanted him to figure it out without me having to say a word. I wanted him to hear my shame through his stethoscope, to detect it in my breathing, to sense it in my heartbeats. I wanted him to see the signs and come to the right conclusion. But my silence left him no choice but to send me home with a name for what I had and a cure should it happen again. It was called hyperventilating, and should it happen again, I was to grab a paper bag and breathe in and out of it as if it were a balloon.

It turned out that the only thing wrong with me was that I was suffering from a temporary lack of oxygen.

Chapter 16

We were embarking on the trip of a lifetime, driving all the way from Petersburg, Ontario, to Charlottetown, Prince Edward Island, stopping along the way to see my Uncle Stan and Aunt Ginger in Halifax. I was excited about the trip. The Maritimes seemed to be a far away and exotic place. I pictured the lobster traps and the lighthouses, Peggy's Cove, Anne of Green Gables. We'd drive the distance dragging the tent trailer behind us. It was packed and loaded, done the night before, already hooked up to Dad's car. Our trailer was not a palace, but it was spacious and fit the three of us nicely. Its single room served as kitchen, dining room, sitting room, and bedroom (sleeping six comfortably, three beautifully). There was even a toilet and shower. The whole contraption folded to look no bigger than a flatbed trailer. But when it was time to set things up, the metal top rose to become a roof, the canvas walls expanded on metal supports and hinges that pulled out at the sides and the front, lengthening, heightening, and widening the trailer in all directions. For the next few weeks, our home would be on wheels. And for the next few weeks we would be a family that travelled together. Mom, Dad, JoJo (our new dog, a small black terrier/poodle mix), and me — always in sight of each other.

We were in the trailer. I was reading my *Archie* comics instead of the cool superhero comics that I should be reading. But I was going through a real Betty and Veronica stage. Mostly Betty. I bought into the comic's portrayal of Veronica as a spoiled, rich, self-interested vixen and Betty as the sweet girl next door. I was lying on the fold-out bed that was not yet pushed back into the shape of a couch. Mom was out, just for a moment and not so far away that she couldn't be seen, and yet Dad was there lying beside me. A chance not taken is an opportunity missed. Perhaps this would be the kind of lesson a father should teach his son, but in the hands of my father, the lesson and the method were questionable.

Mom could return at any moment. I could see Dad glance out the trailer window watching Mom draping damp towels over a makeshift clothesline. I had begun sketching Betty and Veronica when Dad came over, and my drawing piqued his interest. Or so was his reason this time.

He slid onto the cushions beside me, like a playmate squeezing in to see what game I was playing, the venetian blind window in the front of the trailer now at eye level. A perfect view of my mother outside in the campsite. He could do what he wanted. I wouldn't call out, I wouldn't cry for help, get my mother's attention. I was more terrified of being caught than he was. How that happened left me confused, bewildered, and guilty. I had been successfully converted into the villain. Time was my only option for escape — time when he finally grew tired of this game, of me, or when I just grew up and left the home. Surely the grip on me was not so strong as to moor me to him forever. But there was that fear.

He was quiet. Watching Mom, negotiating the risk factor, watching me. I withdrew as much as I could, but the limited space in a camper trailer didn't offer a lot. I focused even harder on my sketch. Hoping, as I always did, that he would acknowledge that I was busy. That I wasn't available. A ludicrous expectation for me to have, given the reality of past transgressions — my availability did not matter. I then tried to lose myself in the drawing, not into the picture as if it were some comic book portal that would land me in Pop's soda shop or Miss Grundy's Riverdale High classroom — if that were possible, I'd have done it long ago — but to lose myself in the act of drawing. I wanted to be invisible, but no matter how faint I made my presence, he would always see me.

"I'm drawing free-hand," I said, taking pride in how accurate the reproductions of the characters were. That was always there, the need to please him, to win his favour, to show him all that I was able to achieve — always a delusional hope that perhaps this time he really was interested in what I was doing. But, even then, I knew better. My body tensed the closer he shifted alongside me. During each encounter — this one included — I became a stone, neither moving nor allowing any participation other than the things forced upon me: the movement of my hand to his genitals, the demands he made, and still I stayed the unenergized, docile partner. A life-like puppet responding only in ways that nature dictated. He gave my drawings a cursory glance then looked at the comic book.

"I want to see how you draw them." He pointed to a panel in the comic book featuring both Betty and Veronica in profile. I showed him a shoulders-up sketch of Betty, smiling her perfect American girl smile.

"No these," he said, indicating the girl's breasts. He caressed the image. I shouldn't have been bothered by these acts of his, not any longer, but he was a man constantly capable of pushing against new boundaries, so that he couldn't even look at a kid's comic book without making it sexual. My dad was aroused by comic book boobs. My dad found a way to make the Archies lewd and provocative.

I hated the callous dismissal of my drawings. I wasn't interested in taking them where he wanted me to go, so I didn't. Not just out of an act of defiance, but for practical reasons as well. Nothing was going to happen since Mom was just outside the trailer. So, I got up, packed my comics, and moved to the other side of the trailer. Twenty feet away. Away from groping hands. I might not be able to protect myself, but I sure as hell could protect Betty and Veronica.

The trailer tilted slightly as Mom stepped onto the black metal stairs. All traces of what almost happened disappeared like a shadow beneath a flood of light. I had perfected an ability to not just hide, but to completely obliterate any wrongdoing. To switch from bad to good at the first sound of a doorhandle turning.

I was already lost in thought when Mom stepped inside. The Archie comic put back in its place; Betty and Veronica's breasts no longer exposed. My drawings untainted.

"It's warming up," Mom said, pulling the door closed with a satisfying click of the bolt latching into the strike plate.

"Put on a sweater." Dad's solution to everything. All the world's ailments could be solved by slipping into a cardigan.

"Why would I put on a sweater when I just said it's warming up?"

"Because it's still cool out there. I'm cold."

"Then you put on a sweater. I'm not cold."

"How could you not be cold?" Dad was unable to conceive that people could possibly experience something different than him.

The sweater conversation — it wasn't an argument — could have been lobbed back and forth until Mom gave in or Dad gave up. The repeated use of the word *sweater* brought images of Betty and Veronica back to mind, and I couldn't tune them out. It was time to go outside. I got up from the folded-out table — one that could collapse into a bed. I was a few inches from the door when Dad smelled something. We were three people in a twenty-five-foot trailer: odours were bound to happen.

"Something stinks," Dad said.

"I don't smell anything, Clare," Mom said.

"You can't smell that?" Dad was looking at me but talking to Mom.

I didn't smell anything, but I knew that would hardly matter. Dad smelled it. Time to leave before things got worse. I couldn't get to my jacket. I couldn't get to the door. Mom was beside me trying to detect the phantom smell, and Dad was beside her. The two of them barring my escape.

Dad's eyes were fixed on me. He's agitated but there was also a hint of mischief, like someone relishing the fact that they're setting you up for a fall. He looked at my running shoes sitting by the door, properly aligned, side by side, out of anyone's way, but sadly, not out of view. "It's your shoes."

He's right. I'd been wearing those runners for some time now. But I was a kid, so I did what kids did in situations like that. I denied it.

"I don't smell anything," I said, which was true, because God knows I've acclimatized to the smell of my own feet. Neither Mom nor I moved, unsure of where this was heading. Bad smells have the potential for comedy. Was this a funny bad smell or was something else about to happen?

"You don't smell anything?" Dad's voice now suggested less humour, but I left the option open. "Yeah. It's his shoes." He brought Mom in. If this was to go south, there would be no hope of Mom having my back.

"It could be. I don't smell anything either," said Mom. It was the sweater argument all over again, redirected at me.

"Give me those," he demanded.

"Oh yeah, it's his shoes," said Mom, tossing off the comment to defuse the situation. Stinky feet were funny, right? I know what you're trying to do, Mom, but no, not helping.

"Give me them." His voice stern, his face a flush of red. Jokes were no longer welcomed. My "this is nothing to raise such a stink over" comment would have to wait for another day.

"Give them!" he shouted again. My mother went silent. I handed the shoes over. "It's your shoes," he said, satisfied that the accusation had been confirmed. Mystery solved, and for a moment it seemed as if he regained composure. I would take my shoes outside, and we could get on with this wonderful family road trip.

Uh-huh. And he can take you fishing, maybe toss a ball around, teach you the proper way to start a campfire. Endless possibilities. It was disconcerting that the Wild Boy was reclining on the still opened-as-a-bed couch, flipping through a comic I thought I had properly stored away. I had been managing fine without him.

Dad held the shoe like a grenade about to explode

"You've stunk up the whole place. What are they doing in here? You keep your stinking shoes outside. You think we want to smell your feet all day? What's the matter with you?" Dad's anger grew like a distant rolling thunder. And just as the size of a trailer can amplify the stench from a pair of running shoes, so can it amplify the heat from an angry man's rage.

He took a step. The fabric of his shirt brushed my chin as he reached for the copper knob of the trailer door. A twist and a push, the metal door swung open, wide and fast enough to extend beyond its springs, banging against the trailer side and back again. The door's return threw Dad's momentum off, turning his fury into a stumbling comic mess.

There is always that, isn't there? The sight gag of your dad being angry.

He pushed the door open again and flung my shoes outside. One and then the next, nearly hitting the trailer beside us.

"Your feet stink, too," he said. "Don't you wash them?" A whole new hell had begun. I wasn't sure what to do. My mother stood to one side. I was close enough for her to step in between us. He'd hit me, but he wouldn't hit her. At least, I'd never seen my father hit my mother. I doubt he did. But there were plenty of secrets in our house.

Things happened quickly. So, if there was no time for me to react, I assume there was no time for her to react. If I couldn't see what was coming next, how could I have expected her to?

She's your mother. There were two kids before you. She's seen this before. She's supposed to anticipate danger. That's what mothers do. Why let her off the hook? You think because you're adopted that the connection a birth mother has with her child doesn't apply to you?

He gripped my arm in one hand and yanked me toward him. I was thrown off balance, tipping slightly as I struggled to regain my footing. I brushed past my mother. She stepped out of the way. I think I saw her almost raise a hand to help, or maybe it was just to prevent me from crashing into her. His other hand grabbed at my shirt. He wanted to shake me, he wanted to throw me, he wanted me out of his sight.

It's the Betty and Veronica drawing, you know. Surprised you didn't just draw their tits. Let him feel you up a bit. Isn't that what you usually do? I thought you had a system?

The trailer rocked, squeaking on its coils as he struggled to shove me out the door. Ironic, since I was also struggling to get out the door. From the outside it must have seemed like a barroom brawl had broken out. I was facing him when he finally had me positioned in the frame of the open door. He shoved me out, still yelling. I stumbled down the black metal stairs, my momentum carrying me backward until I fell on the ground — very close to my shoes. He stood in the doorway yelling at me to stay outside. To get lost. Mom watched. She was telling me to leave. I could hardly hear her. I could only hear and see my dad. I would have preferred to have been angry, but I could only work up the strength to be scared.

The trailer door shut. No satisfying click. Just sudden silence.
I stayed down for a while. I put on my shoes. They did stink.

I stood. It had been raining. There was mud and grass on my hands. I was afraid I was going to start crying. So, what if I did? Who was there to see me? It was a Monday. There were trailers everywhere, but they were locked. If there was anyone here, they were holed up inside, safe behind aluminum doors. Perhaps no one heard. Perhaps everyone heard. Perhaps no one thought it mattered. I was twelve. Crowded places with no one there to help were everywhere. I'd become used to it.

I headed away from the trailer. There was a wooded area nearby. I had come across it the day before. It took me by surprise when the woods opened into a large field, and there in the field was a two-seater plane. Seeing something so big, so unexpected took my breath away. This was where I went because I wanted to be astounded again. I wanted to be overwhelmed by something remarkable.

I wanted to run away like kids in movies run away from their mean guardians, from cruel aunts and uncles, from workhouses and orphanages. How mean did a parent have to be before running away could be considered heroic? I thought about what happened at the trailer. Was it violent or was it trivial? I didn't think being yelled at for having stinky feet would count as run-away mean. They fed me. They clothed me. They bought me presents at Christmas and on my birthday. They took me with them on camping vacations. And there were plenty of days when they were kind.

I imagined the commotion that would follow when they discovered I was gone. Mom would start looking for me, calling out my name, angry, wondering where the hell had I gone off to this time. In time, Dad would join the search to make two angry parents searching for their delinquent kid. Eventually the police would have to be called. I wonder if fear would start to set in then and what kind of fear it would be. Would they be fearful of my whereabouts and welfare, or would they be fearful for what the police might discover if I were found?

Then there'd be the search parties, photocopied missing person posters on grocery store bulletin boards and hydro poles, items on the local news. And what would be said when I was found? The police would hear about my father getting angry over my stinky running shoes and kicking me out of the trailer. I could see them look at each other, I could see the faces of the people in the search party laughing. I imagined morning news anchors joking about the boy who ran away because his feet stank. I could see the embarrassment and shame on my parents' faces. And when word got out that I was adopted, they would say, "He's lucky to have parents when there are so many children out there without a mother and a father."

So, I waited where I was, looking at the airplane in the open field. I waited until I was less angry. Waited until I got hungry, until the light began to fade. I waited until it was time for me to go back home.

Dad was right. I did need a sweater.

Chapter 17

I can't accuse the Wild Boy of pushing an anti-Christian agenda on me, but I also can't say that he wasn't without influence. I was watching a Christian television talk show. The on-air preacher was doing one of those miraculous reaching-out-through-the-television-screen to see his viewers — a trick utilized best, I think, in early episodes of *Romper Room*. The Wild Boy didn't disapprove of my watching these shows, and I doubt he'd have told me if he did. I knew he didn't agree with what was being said, and he was never in any danger of being converted; he just saw them as entertaining. He'd laugh a lot during them. Not me. I still held out for a miracle.

"I feel there is someone out there watching right now who needs the healing touch of Jesus," said the television evangelist.

Wild Boy laughed. He leaned into me. *Do you think he's talking about you?* he asked.

My goodness, I thought, he is. He is talking about me. There you go. At least Jesus knows.

The studio where the evangelist sat speaking to his faceless congregation seemed sparse. Not even the magic of television could alter the makeshift garage-studio look. A single desk in the centre of the screen, the evangelist staring straight into the camera while the disembodied voice of a late-night caller in need of salvation struggled to get through another night. They prayed, and then, with a new soul bound to the spirit of Christ, the phone line was cleared. That's when Jesus called out to me again.

"There is someone out there right now. Jesus is sending me your pain. You feel like everyone has deserted you. You're lost. The Devil wants you to stay lost. But Jesus wants you found. He's waiting for your call."

I thought it best not to keep Jesus waiting. The Wild Boy must have thought so, too. Not that he had any great faith in J.C.'s healing powers, he just understood that Jesus was in high demand and would move on if we didn't act quickly. Wild Boy dialed the phone number that appeared at the bottom of the television screen and held the receiver out me. I heard the distinct sound of a broadcast-studio ring. I placed the receiver to my ear, waited for a few more rings before someone answered.

"Thank you for calling, how may Jesus help you?" The voice at the other end of the line belonged to a woman. It was not the voice of the determined-looking evangelist who was now busy praying over the airwaves with another lost soul. My intent was to be polite: "Yes. Good evening. I'm hoping you can connect me to the proper person who deals with young boys being sexually abused by their fathers? ... Yes, I can hold." But all polite intent left when I heard the woman's officious and, what I interpreted to be, judgmental tone. It was as if someone had managed to fill an entire bucket with every ounce of my anger, and then dumped it over my head. All those nights I came to God, trusting prayer to be the answer. *Please make this stop*, I prayed. Prayed that my father would no longer want to play this game. I begged for forgiveness for letting it go on. I begged to be forgiven for allowing it to feel good. I prayed that whatever I was doing to tempt my father and lead him astray would stop. I was sorry for not being better at sports, not being more interested in hockey. I was sorry that I talked so much, and for loving movies, and for writing and reading. I was sorry for not being the boy my father had wanted me to be. But my prayers were ignored. And now I had the chance to ask why God decided to turn his head and look the other way.

If I couldn't be polite than I could at least be curt, to the point, and professional. "Yes. Hello. I'm being sexually abused by my dad, and I keep praying to God to make it stop but he hasn't. So, I'm calling to find out why God's been ignoring my prayers."

The woman on the other line was silent. I assumed she was collecting her thoughts, trying to format a proper, sensitive but pro-God response. She wasn't.

"Are you accusing God of not caring?" she asked. I didn't have a lot of experience in upsetting adults, but I think I could comfortably say that she was alarmed.

"No, no," I corrected, still drenched in anger, but not willing to alienate my chance of a televised debate, "I just think he's not listening."

"I assure you God hears every prayer." The on-air conversation between television preacher and current caller leaked in through the earpiece. I wondered if the woman I was talking to was in the same room. Could he hear parts of our conversation, too?

Tell her he didn't seem to hear yours.

"Well, he didn't seem to hear mine." I nodded to the Wild Boy, thanking him for his input. It was the kind of wise rebuttal that usually doesn't come to me until much later.

"Did you let it happen? What have you done to stop it?" the woman asked.

I didn't like the question, but it was me who called her, not her who called me, so it was only fair that I answered.

"I was scared. I was afraid of what he might do. And I didn't want to tell anyone. I didn't want anyone finding out."

Say this: Besides, if I talk to God, I don't need to talk to anyone else. Right? Because God's all powerful and he loves children and stuff. I put a finger in my ear to block out the Wild Boy.

"Well, of course you didn't want anyone finding out. You're a boy. Why didn't you fight back? How old are you now?"

How old am I now? Didn't want to answer that either. And I was still considering how I should respond to the "You're a boy, why didn't you fight back?" question. Well, yes. Yes, I am a boy. Thank you. But you see, I'm one of those boys who enjoys writing, reading, and watching movies, so, fighting's not really something I do.

"I'm almost thirteen," I lied. I was almost fourteen, but I was afraid if she knew that, she'd hang up.

"Thirteen? Why didn't you fight back when you were twelve?"

Why twelve? Is twelve some magical number where boys were suddenly capable of beating up their abusive fathers? Is that the age boys were suddenly free from the grip that years of abuse, abusive training, and brainwashing had on them?

"I'd like to speak to the host," I said, but my adolescent voice lacked the conviction it needed to register with the woman on the phone. She told me that wasn't going to happen but that she would pray with me.

"I did pray. I prayed and prayed and prayed and prayed. And God did nothing. That's why I'm calling. I want to know why God did not answer my prayers."

"God helps those who help themselves," she said. "You should have fought back."

The Wild Boy whispered this into my ear — *Tell her she knows nothing about sexual abuse.*

"You know nothing about child sexual abuse, do you?" I told the woman.

The woman took my insult in stride. "You need to pray. You need to bring Christ into your life," she said.

And you need to be better educated before you think you can start doling out advice on helplines, whispered the Wild Boy.

"And you need to be better educated before you think you can start doling out advice on helplines," I said.

Now hang up.

And I hung up. The Wild Boy seemed pleased.

At least we know that God is not an option, the Wild Boy said, smiling.

* * *

I was fourteen. I made it out of junior high and into high school simply by living one day as it bled into the next. I manoeuvred through the neighbourhood, in and out of school, waging minor struggles for my independence where I could. I earned pocket money working with Gerry Stoltz who took over Montag's farm after they became too old to farm anymore. I also had a part-time job at Knechtle's, the local grocery store. Dennis worked there. He became a star employee at Knechtle's and a top student at Waterloo-Oxford High. Our friendship never recovered from the grade six fallout when Dennis led a campaign to ostracize me from our friend group. We talked now and then. We were courteous, but Dennis stayed aloof, kept the upper hand, and he always found something about me — or Doug — to scorn. Basically, Dennis just grew up faster than the rest of us. Faster than me.

Dad was impatient with my lack of progress through puberty. There was no physical difference between who I was at fourteen and who I was at twelve, except for maybe height.

This was not just an issue for my dad, but it became an issue socially. I was in high school. Waterloo-Oxford. It was mandatory to take a shower after gym class. Our gym teacher was — get this — my cousin Wayne. Dad's nephew. He sat at the entrance to the boys' shower and marked who did and who didn't take a shower. Nothing weird, just assuring that personal hygiene was adhered to. If you don't shower you failed the class, and so I became the only kid I knew of who managed to fail gym class. But how could I have stood in front of my classmates, naked and ashamed of my hairless, undeveloped, tarnished body? The legacy of my dad's abuse had begun revealing itself in corners of my life that I thought would always be protected.

Dad also questioned why I wasn't ejaculating yet, although he did say he could tell when I was *done* by the way my body tensed. He didn't know how that tense feeling was more pain than pleasure. It was too much. It was too intense. It was like being stabbed in the abdomen or jolted with a live wire.

My go-to sexual fantasy was to imagine the scene from the book *Northwest Passion* where the "sultry" brunette seduces the "sweet," innocent blond in the front seat of the car. It's an odd fantasy because I'm not even in it. I fantasize, too, about Emma Peel from reruns of *The Avengers*. It helps that her last name is *Peel* and she wears a skin-tight black leather jumpsuit. That fantasy mostly involves peeling her out of her skin-tight jumpsuit.

I met Diana hitchhiking along Highway 8 in front of our house. She saw me watching her, crossed the road, and started walking toward me even though about five cars, which might very well have stopped for her, drove by. I figured she was mad that I was staring at her, but I would tell her, when I got the chance, that I meant nothing by it — just curiosity from seeing someone my age who I hadn't seen before. Her gaze was fixed on me like she'd lose track of where I was standing if she were to look away. Turned out she wasn't mad, just hot and thirsty. She wanted a drink. Could I give her one?

Mom and Dad weren't home, so I told her to wait outside while I went in and got her a glass of water. Diana had been hitchhiking since the outskirts of Kitchener, walking the whole time without so much as a car slowing down.

I figured Diana to be a year or so older than me — fifteen, maybe.

She took the glass of water and drank it without pause. She really was thirsty.

She said she lived in a group home in St. Agatha, told me she had a bit of a reputation for being a "bad" girl. Did I like bad girls, or did I like girls who go to church and stuff?

"I don't know," I said.

She smiled. "But you do like girls?"

"Sure."

"Good." She said she needed a break from hitchhiking and wouldn't mind hanging out for a while.

I didn't find Diana particularly attractive. She lacked a softness that I think would have appealed to me at the time. Maybe I did prefer church girls. But I wanted her to stay. I wanted her to keep looking at me the way she did. I wanted to hear more about what it was like to be a bad girl.

"We'll hang out," I told her. "You want another glass of water?"

"No. So, what's there to do around here?"

"I dunno. There's a bridge back behind the house that goes over the railway track. We could go there."

"Is it far?"

"Nah, just down the laneway, behind the barn."

"Okay." The smile again.

Diana liked the bridge crossing the railway tracks. She said it was peaceful and if she lived here, the bridge was where she'd spend all her time. We sat together with our legs hanging over the side waiting for the train to pass. We counted the cars as the train passed along the rails beneath us.

When Diana asked me if I ever kissed a girl, I said, "Plenty of times," and to prove it, I leaned in and pecked her on the cheek.

"What was that?" she said. "Is that how you kiss your grandmother?"

"I don't have a grandmother," I told her. "I'm adopted."

"You're lucky," she said. "Here," she grabbed the back of my head with one hand and pulled me toward her lips. She kept me there with our lips pressed together. She opened her mouth. I was afraid she was going to bite me — one of those erotic nips piercing the flesh of my lip that I read about in *Northwest Passion* — but instead her tongue glided inside my mouth. I didn't know what it was, at first, and wanted to pull away, but the sensation of it was strangely satisfying. Soon my hand was reaching up to hold her head, not wanting her to leave, not wanting to break whatever spell was washing over me.

"You can touch me," she said, "but just on the outside. And only on top."

Fair enough. I touched her, though I wasn't sure what exactly I was supposed to do or even why I should want to do it. My head was still in the kiss. I felt as if I might topple off the bridge and onto the tracks. After a while, Diana pulled away from me, smiling again.

"You're funny," she said and stood up. "Come on. I have to be back, or I'll be in deep shit."

Deep shit? Wow, she is a bad girl.

Whatever I did that was funny was a good funny because she held my hand for the entire walk back to my place. Mom and Dad were getting out of the car just as we arrived. Diana went over and introduced herself, a move that seemed suspiciously like someone covering up a bad deed. She wasted no time telling them that she was hitchhiking and how nice I was to offer her a glass of cold water. The empty glass still stood on the front steps as evidence.

Mom and Dad looked at me to see if there was anything else that needed to be said, that Diana hadn't bothered mentioning. I just stared at my feet.

"You were hitchhiking by yourself?" Mom asked her, already forming an opinion of a young girl who dared to hitchhike on her own. "Where are you going?"

"St. Agatha." And then, "To a group home."

Mom nodded as if that explained everything.

"I'll give you a lift," Dad said. Mom said that's a better idea than having her continue hitchhiking. It's not safe for a girl to hitchhike alone. She would go, too.

Diana didn't hesitate in accepting and wondered if I would come, too. I didn't. I made up an excuse about having to finish something. No one questioned me. What I needed was to go to my room, keep Diana's kiss in mind, remember it as if she were still with me, to recall the feel of her breasts in my hands.

I didn't see Diana again, at least not in person, but she returned frequently in my fantasies — quick and obscene. Diana was my bad girl fantasy. My good girl fantasy was a girl called Laurel Mitchell. The Wild Boy preferred Diana. And although I could appreciate Diana, my crush on Laurel took me to a different place — something I imagined to be love. It lasted through high school.

Laurel Mitchell was a reserved but popular ginger-haired classmate. I saw in her a soft, warm, and unattainable affection. I thought she could save me. She couldn't, of course, so my fantasy was never her saving me, but me saving her. And in that fantasy, I was a different boy than I was. In my fantasy, I'm kind and virtuous. I'm untarnished and brave. I'm strong and confident.

In the Laurel Mitchell fantasy, I'd rescued her from some evil person who meant her harm and I was taking her back home to her parents. But it had become dark, and it was too late to go any farther. We found a wooded enclosure, safe among a cloister of trees. I started a small fire that kept us warm. I comforted her and assured her that she was safe with me and would be home soon. And then we kissed. I was more startled by the kiss than she was. It was a wonderful and sweet kiss, powerful enough to break both our hearts. When I went to hold her, she asked me to hold her even harder. And we laid down on the pine needles and in the grass, wrapped in each other's arms, and the overwhelming feeling that came from the warmth of our bodies was more beauty than anyone could ever need.

But the fantasy always left me feeling guilty. I knew that if Laurel ever needed help, she wouldn't seek it from me. And as far as the Wild Boy knew, Diana might have thought herself to be a bad girl, but what are the chances that she was? These were just things the Wild Boy and I imagined and had hoped for. And yet, there was nothing in our fantasies with either Laurel or Diana that could be found in the pages of *Northwest Passion*. And there was nothing like our imagined love for them in any of my dad's descriptions of what it was like to be with a woman. Even the Wild Boy appreciated that.

Chapter 18

- - - - - - - - - -

It began when Mom went to the hospital. It started in the living room in a chair that now looks to me like a devil's throne with bad upholstery and the ability to recline. And on that chair Dad sat, perched like a spoiled, lustful king ruled by the whims of his most basic desires, calling me over so I could hop onto his lap and play his little tickle game. That's when it started. Somewhere then at the age of seven or eight or nine or ten. I recall so many events that fall in between then and now: Wasaga Beach, the drive-ins, the public showers at the trailer park, reading segments from *Northwest Passion*, him wanting to "try something new," coming into my bedroom between periods in the hockey game, making sure to be back at the television before the start of the next period — a good Leafs game trumps everything. Who knows how things might have been had the Leafs been a better team? Of all these things, only a few have a time or a date, and they are not necessarily remembered in the right order. Instead, they sit in my memory like apples in a bushel.

But I know when it ended. Unequivocally. August 1975. I was seventeen. Puberty had finally caught up to me. I was practically an adult. I was of the age of consent. This could no longer be called child abuse but compliant incest. But for eight, or nine, or ten years I'd been groomed to respond to his demands without thought or resistance. If it didn't stop then, would it have stopped at all?

My summer that year was spent in Red Lake. Red Lake was about as far north as you could get and still be in Ontario. Mom sent me there. She got wind of this Junior Forest Rangers program where seventeen-year-old boys — there's one for seventeen-year-old girls, too, but the paths between boys and girls never cross — work a summer at a provincial park maintaining campsites, forging fire trails, fighting fires if necessary — or at least that was the sell on the brochure. There were things the brochure probably didn't mention: military brush cuts and uniformed outfits, early morning calisthenics and bunking in a barracks with a crew of late night masturbators and early morning farters.

This was not part of my summer plans. Not that my plans went beyond working at Knechtle's grocery store and a bit at Stoltz's farm, hanging out at Val and Wayne's pool, babysitting Dave and Denny, going to drive-ins, catching a few summer blockbusters, maybe do a camping trip of my own. But Mom had other ideas. Forms were filled, train tickets bought, suitcase packed, and I was ready to leave before I even knew what was going down. "No if ands or buts," Mom said. "I'm not having you sit around on your duff all summer. Like it or not you're going." This made me determined to hate it even more. After all, I was growing my hair long, I was slowly gaining ground on my independence, though much of this was fallacy, for I was still enslaved by the whims and desires of my dad.

Turns out Junior Forest Rangers had a lot to offer, like a molestation-free summer for one thing, the first in a decade. (It was such a new freedom for me that I didn't masturbate once that entire summer — a record, I bet, for any seventeen-year-old boy.)

Dad wasn't happy the day I left. He lost his temper with me at the train station, like he was jealous or something, like I was getting married too young, to a Catholic. Luckily, Uncle Quinnie was with us, so even though things got embarrassing, they didn't get violent. But something happened during the summer. Something to make my parents pack up and leave their precious rural life, move into the city, which they said would never happen, and immerse themselves in a new devotion to Christ by joining a church that demanded every word in the Bible be taken literally. All these changes in the two months I was away, and except for the boxes of photographs and dusty memorabilia, everything was unpacked and in place by the time I got home. So, something happened, but no one was talking.

It didn't strike me as strange at the time. If it had, then maybe I'd have done some investigating, asked a few questions, gone back to the neighbourhood to find out what set this sudden change of events into motion. But how could I possibly see anything as strange? How could a boy, now a young man, whose sex life began at the hands of his father, long before he reached puberty, and continued well through his teens — how could that boy determine what was strange? How could anything seem unnatural, irregular, mysterious, out-of-sorts, not-quite-right, bizarre, peculiar, questionable, when the most unnatural, unbelievable atrocity had become part of my norm? No, that boy — me — would not think such a dramatic change of lifestyle and beliefs unusual at all. Like everything else, things were just the way they were. I now lived in the city, my parents no longer drank, or danced, or read unless it was the Bible, and — the most important change of all — we now owned a colour television.

I had changed, too. I had conquered the past and had control of the future. The summer gave me a belief in who I was and who I could be, a belief that the moment I hoped and longed for had finally arrived. And though I feared my body might still betray me,

I felt as if a corner had been turned. I came back home confident that my old life was over.

But here I was again, lying with my born-again Christian father who was taking a break from highlighting passages in the Bible, and all the progress I made over the summer left me. I couldn't defy him. I didn't even try.

And then the end begins.

"What are we doing?" Dad shouted, the words coming out with incredulous disdain, an attack of the conscience, as if he had woken from a thirty-year nightmare and found his son had crawled naked into bed with him. Like Adam and Eve suddenly aware of their nakedness. So now not only had he robbed me of my youth, of my right to discover and develop my own sexuality, robbed me of a father, of a childhood, he was robbing me of the right to wake up from this nightmare, the nightmare he was waking up from. The fucker. That moment belongs to me.

"Get out!" he screamed. But my body, my mind, my thoughts couldn't comprehend the words coming out of his mouth. They had no context. Not here. Not in this situation. Words so far removed from what I'd been trained, taught, and come to expect now had no meaning. I had spent years upon years upon years on the other side of those words. But as my words they had no strength. My words could only plead, beg, negotiate, and only on one occasion had they been threatening.

"Get out!" he screamed again, and I tried to move because I knew too well how quickly the monster takes over. But I didn't get out fast enough. My body had grown strong over the summer, capable of fighting back, capable of crashing down on him, turning his weakness against him, leaving him broken and bleeding. But my mind was weak. I was still the little boy unable to fight back. I'd been trained to believe that this was my reality and that it could not be changed.

And now his anger — an anger that rightfully belonged to me — was being hurled against me as if all these years I had been the rapist, the molester, the instigator, the tormentor, the manipulator. As though it were I who plotted and groomed him into becoming a child abuser. As though it were I who was the tempter who led this godly man astray and lured him into betrayal and incest. As though the spell that overtook him was cast long before I was born, long before the day that I took his hand in an ice cream store and charmed an entire family into welcoming me in as one of their own.

And then he started kicking me as if I was too unclean to beat with his hands.

It was me who had been the demon all along. His years of groping and touching and playing secret little games were my fault.

What had he seen in my face when the truth of who he was came rushing at him? Did he see my fear, my accusations, my shame? Did they reflect at him so that he saw the same in himself?

How I hoped so. How I hoped that Dad, now proclaiming to be an outspoken champion of Christ, a soldier for the Lord, a guardian of the good word, was struck by the weight and the horror he'd created and came face to face with the evil he'd done. How I hoped for a retribution that would make his soul cave in, leave him weeping and shaking in shame and regret, unable to stand from knowledge of the sheer atrocities of his actions, terrified, beyond shock and pain and remorse. But Dad only had a look of disgust and utter disdain, and the source of his disgust and disdain was me.

I fell to the floor with no clear thought as to what was happening. I managed to push myself up on my elbows, my feet slipping beneath me, not enough space between the bed and the closet to scurry away. There was no way of knowing how far his anger would go. Times before this he was just a pathetic man, but now he had the wrath of God. He was powered with righteous indignation. He was a holy man tortured and humiliated by the lustful lure of youth. How dare I? How I must have looked to him. No longer a child but a man. My body no longer hairless, my muscles formed and shaped. How revolting I must have seemed — the body of a man who submits so easily.

On the day that it ended, I was kicked from the bed, completely naked in front of my dad, lying splayed on the floor like a scorned lover, scrambling to my room for safety, taking on his shame and his blame, believing it to be my own.

Through the kicking and the beating, I was thinking that this was it, this was the end I'd been waiting for. And who knew that it would be him who got to end it? Not me. That power was never going to belong to me, because I was never, and never will be, capable of saving myself.

It was a toss-up as to who found who — did Dad find God or did God find Dad? Presumably, this was the same God who ignored my prayers when, as a child, I went to him in good faith to ask him to save me from abuse, and yet welcomed my father without question or judgment. That God. Or is this what they mean when they talk about God working in mysterious ways? I suppose it could be argued that my prayers were answered. After all, all sexual interaction with Dad stopped the moment after he hurled me from the bed he and his wife shared. But somehow that seemed like his victory, not mine. And in its place, a new persecution began. The religious wars.

Dad became a staunch, solid, Hollywood stereotype of the religious warrior. More cunning than Burt Lancaster in *The Rainmaker*, more malicious than Robert Mitchum in *The Night of the Hunter*, and more self-righteous than Paul Sorvino in *Oh, God!*, Dad's faith rained down like a plague of locusts, prophesying doom, not just for me, but for all his children, his family, and his friends. And at what cost was Dad's salvation? Did he confess his sins to God in front of others? Was he crystal clear on the exact nature of his sins? Or was it a confession made in the privacy of his own thoughts and prayers?

But, of course, God would have already known. Dad wouldn't have had to endure the humiliation of voicing his sins aloud. A simple prayer of forgiveness and Dad was off the hook. Hallelujah!

Dad found God. And through God he discovered how much better of a person he was than everyone else. No longer tempted by the evil seduction of his adopted son, free from drink, from tobacco, and from all earthly vices. He even threw away his copy of *Northwest Passion*. He became a follower of Christ — one of God's foot soldiers. And those who had dared to have turned him against God, who had led him astray with their seductions and desires, they, too, must find the Lord or perish for their sins. And those — mainly me — who polluted their souls with rock music and R-rated movies, those who refused to stand against abortion, condemn Jews, Muslims, Buddhists, Hindus, Mormons, Jehovah's Witnesses, Catholics, soft-sell religions, and atheists as sinners, would one day face the wrath of God.

"I'm proud to be the only one standing up for Christ," Dad loved to say, beaming with the strength of the inner spirit. Mom followed him. Why wouldn't she? She had followed him without question through everything before God, so why not after? She sat with her husband, and they'd underline passages in their Bibles. He had a mission: to save the wretched souls of this lost world, the souls of his children. And so, my father took it upon himself to lead us all onto the path of righteousness. He was our shepherd, our guide, our spiritual leader. He was going to be a father, after all.

And he set his sights on my sister Valerie to be the first recipient of his good graces.

* * *

Dad was at work. He had retired from Uniroyal and took up work as a janitor at a public grade school. Not to worry, he was reformed.

God had stepped in, right? A knock on the door. It was Wayne. This was not to be a social visit, Mom and I both knew. We could tell by the knock, by the hour of the day, by the fact that Wayne was alone.

Mom wiped her hands on her apron and went to the door; there was no smile on her face, only a grimace that was working itself into something similar to a smile. Mom greeted Wayne with a welcoming "what a surprise. How nice to see you," but there was nothing in her voice to suggest that it was nice to see him at all. Wayne stood in the doorway, not coming in, sturdy and unmovable, no warmth in his greeting, none of Wayne's cheerful exuberance but a steely concern and a firm gaze.

"I'm not coming in, Margaret," Wayne said.

I watched from the kitchen. Normally I would greet Wayne at the door, join Mom in welcoming him into the house. It was strange to see him now in the middle of the week without my sister, without the boys.

"What's up?" Mom asked, still feigning optimism. I didn't move any nearer. Mom stepped farther into the door frame, blocking part of Wayne from view. I could see my mother in profile, her eyes in unwavering contact with Wayne's. If an accusation was to be made, then eye contact would be proof of her innocence.

Mom listened to Wayne as he described Dad's impromptu arrival at Valerie's door. He had demanded she turn her life over to Christ, and had left my sister crying, fearful, and angry.

No voices were raised. Wayne did most of the talking. Mom explained that they weren't there to upset anyone.

"Clare is not to come to our house again without an invitation and without me there," Wayne said, his voice firm. "Denny was there ..."

"We didn't know he was there, Wayne, or we never would have —" Mom wasn't able to finish coating over the incident with an explanation.

"Denny had to hear his mother crying and hear Clare yelling at her —"

"Honestly, Wayne. We didn't know Denny was there."

"It doesn't matter if you knew or not, Marg." Wayne's voice edged on frustration. "The point is, we have our own religion. We like it and we do not want to hear that we're wrong, we're going to hell, that we were sinners. We don't want to hear about your church again."

"Well, I'm sorry, Wayne, but Clare is just concerned —"

"Be concerned in your own home, with your own kid, not mine."

I left and went into my room. I lost myself in a television program. I didn't hear the rest of the conversation. I didn't hear Wayne leave. I didn't hear what Mom did after she closed the door and Wayne drove away. But it was apparent that Dad had found a new way to hurt his children in the name of the Lord.

* * *

A few weeks later I got news that Dennis had been walking to Knechtle's, where he still worked, when a car passing on the gravel shoulder hit him head on. Dennis died instantly. The car kept going. And despite our years of disconnect, Dennis's mother asked me to give part of the eulogy. My parents knew Dennis well, but they didn't come to the funeral.

It was at a Catholic church.

Dad's gesture of sympathy over the death of a childhood friend amounted to one observation: "Too bad he died without being saved."

Chapter 19

I was nineteen.

Perhaps I'll be thought of as cruel for what I did next.

It was two years after the abuse ended, and I still feared that people would find out. Prayer was no longer a significant part of my life, ever since that experiment had failed me as a child, but when I did try it, it changed from praying for the abuse to end to praying for the secret to be kept forever. I imagined the terrifying possibility of Dad, grown old and feeble, having lost all sense of place and time, blurting to a room full of people some graphic indiscretion that would expose us both. I prayed, too, that I would never be so foolish as to make the abuse public knowledge, to confess to a therapist, or worse, to write a book. I wanted my past to die, and with it all memory to be erased.

Most of all, I wanted to never hear Dad reference that time again.

But then one Sunday as I was making my escape before being coerced into going to some church event, Mom caught me as I headed out the door. "Your father wants to talk to you downstairs," she said, and left the room before I could execute a proper sigh and roll of my eyes.

What does he want? said the Wild Boy. *Better not be about church because I'm not going.*

I went downstairs. Dad was there, looking uncomfortable. He had a look of sincerity and sadness that I had not seen before. In someone else, to someone else, this might have been touching, and I'd have reached out, made things easier, let him know that I understood that this was tough for him, that I was there. Son to father in a moment of reconciliation. The final scene in a difficult chapter where every character realizes the war has ended and the wounds could start to heal.

Fuck, said the Wild Boy, *I knew we should have left sooner.*

I didn't say hello. I would only acknowledge that I was there, but only out of a perverse obligation to maintain the facade that he was my dad. I stood there. Behind him was a wall of photos. Family pictures, including one awful school picture of me that Dad once tore off the wall screaming, "You look like a girl!" horrified by my long hair and stupid gap-toothed grin. He wasn't entirely wrong — I don't think I looked like a girl, but it was an awful picture. The picture was back up on the wall, but it might have been better if he had succeeded in throwing it away. I looked past him at the picture, wondering how old I was when it was taken, and what thoughts I was burying behind that stupid grin.

"I know ..." Dad started. I could tell he was attempting to summon composure, strengthen the will to say something difficult. Whatever it was going to be, I knew I didn't want to hear it. But I heard it, nonetheless. "I know I haven't been much of a father to you."

And the winner of the world's most understated statement goes to ...

I had to stop the Wild Boy from falling to the floor convulsing in breathless laughter.

Dad continued, "I'm sorry. I promise that from now on I'll be a better father."

All my life, the only thing I truly hated was hearing him use the word *father*.

I was nineteen.

The Wild Boy had felt like laughing. He could. He had that freedom. I did not.

The Wild Boy grew antsy, maybe reading my discomfort, egging me to walk away. *Yeah, yeah, yeah, your dad wasn't much of a father. I knew it before he did. Can we go now?*

It had been two years of pretending nothing had happened, of crushing every impulse that would convince me otherwise, that my lucky-to-be-adopted childhood was not just wheelbarrow rides and pushes on the swing.

It had ended. It was done. And so should be the memory.

But then his apology came: insufficient, self-serving, and far too late.

All those years of telling me not to say a thing.

Don't tell. He had said it with fingers pressing against my throat. *Don't tell.*

He had said it time and time again.

Don't tell.

Don't tell.

Don't tell.

But he was telling me. And the shame that brewed just below the surface of my skin, burst through.

So, I could say ... what? *It's okay, Dad. We all make mistakes.* No. That wasn't what he wanted to hear. What he wanted to hear — what I know he wanted to hear — was *don't worry. I'm as much to blame as you are.* And nothing less than that would have been enough. And then we would fall to our knees, weeping and begging for God's forgiveness.

I wish I could say that I felt compassion while watching Dad swallow his pride, struggle through to an apology, standing in front of me, vulnerable, admitting he was wrong. And me, I shuffled my feet, averted my eyes, sighed impatiently, and waited for his stupid confession to end.

Tell him to go fuck yourself off — and see what he does, suggested the Wild Boy.

Instead, I said, "Don't worry about it," and turned my back, abandoning Dad in the basement. Left him there without the satisfaction of a Hallmark moment, no reunion, no embrace, no forgiveness. But he must have taken my words to heart because, as far as I could tell, Dad never did worry about it again.

Not long after that I did what I had hoped I would never do. I told someone. It wasn't planned. It wasn't thought through. It happened. And when it did, even the Wild Boy could only throw up his arms and back away.

I met Valerie at the Fredrick Mall near the home I shared with my parents. Fredrick Mall had a duplex theatre that programmed movies that no one wanted to see — *Cuba, The Fish That Saved Pittsburgh*, and a Scientology-produced propaganda piece starring Gregory Peck — but now they were screening *The Big Chill*, a movie I wanted Valerie to see. After the movie, I suggested we go for a drink, but Valerie, as she will tell you, never learned how to drink. And to be honest, at nineteen, neither had I. We went to the bar and ordered a coffee.

We talked about the movie. Valerie updated me on the kids, both in high school. David had started dating.

And then for no ascertainable reason, nothing that I could look back on and say for certain that that was the reason I blurted out everything I vowed to keep secret, I said, "Do you remember when Mom was in the hospital?"

"Yeah," Valerie said. She must have known something was coming, but I don't think she expected what she heard.

I told Valerie about the armchair where Dad sat and called me onto his lap, I told her about the Hot Wheels car Al had bought for me that Dad wanted a closer look at, I told her about the tickling and about the book *Northwest Passion*. I told her everything. I told her without flinching.

I was nineteen and for the first time I was talking. My words fell out calmly, matter-of-factly. She met me eye-to-eye, heard every word. She didn't shift uncomfortably or try to change the subject. She looked at me while I talked. And when I was done, she looked down into her coffee. We were both silent. Then Valerie waved over the waiter and ordered a drink. She ordered two. She ordered wine. What did I want? A beer.

"What exactly did he do to you?" she asked.

I shrugged. "Stuff."

She shook her head.

"Did he …?" She stopped. Maybe she was afraid of the answer. I knew what she meant. "He tried. But no."

She leaned back, never taking her eyes off me as if trying to contemplate the years of knowing me, of being with me, of being with him, and through all that unaware of what had been happening. Trying to comprehend the when and the where.

"How long did this …?"

"It started when Mom went into the hospital. How old was I then? Seven? Eight? Nine?"

An audible breath out, as if she had been holding it in the whole time. The waiter came with her wine, my beer. He placed the drinks in front of us, asked for my identification, an age of majority card, which, even during this conversation, I happily dug out of my wallet, eager to prove that I had earned the right to drink. The waiter, who reminded me vaguely of someone I had gone to high school with, looked at the government-issued card, compared the photo to me, nodded, smiled, and returned the card. Valerie held the stem of her wine glass — an inexpensive rosé. I don't recall her drinking. Holding a drink seemed to be enough for her. She peered into her glass staring at something visible only to her; a past, perhaps, that she was no longer able to believe in, or a truth she could not comprehend. Had I been careless, too insensitive in blurting out what had to have been a heartbreaking revelation about the man who raised her? Was I too confident that she wouldn't be looking for ways to find me at fault?

We sat like that, saying nothing, long enough that I considered reneging on my confession, as I had with Doug so many years earlier. Then Valerie started to nod, slowly as if coming to life after a long stint of absolute stillness.

"Yeah," Valerie said, still staring into her glass. "It happened to me, too."

It was my turn to show restraint. But unlike my sister, my restraint was strengthened by alcohol. I took a large gulp from my beer.

"Did Mom know?"

"I told her, and she stopped it." I allowed what she said to sit with me. And then she added, "I was five."

Such is the way with secrets; you reveal one to find an even bigger secret beneath.

"He lied," I said. "I asked him if he ever did this with you and Anna. He said he didn't. He was adamant about it. He acted like I was insane to even ask."

"Well, he did. To me, anyway."

"Anna?"

"No," Valerie said.

I consider this. New information to process. Valerie, me, but not Anna.

"How often?"

"Twice. And then I told Mom."

"And she stayed with him."

Valerie shrugs. "It was a different time. Dad was back from the war."

"Dad was never in the war."

"The service. Mom had me, and Anna was on the way."

"He didn't do any fighting. Don't make him into a war hero. He was stationed as a peacekeeper in England after the war where all he did was sleep around with British girls and eat Fig Newtons."

"He told you that?" She meant the sleeping around. We all knew about the Fig Newtons.

"He did."

"Does Mom know?"

"I never told her."

"That would kill her."

"That would kill her, but her five-year-old daughter getting molested didn't?" Valerie investigates her wine glass. Still not drinking. "He tried to strangle me once."

"Man, we have a crazy father."

I wish I had told her that *we* don't have a crazy father, *she* had a crazy father. And I wasn't exactly buying that he was crazy, either. Crazy didn't describe it. Crazy was a dad who goes off on whims and tangents. Crazy could be embarrassing, sometimes funny, worthy of our patience and caring. The word I liked, the word I thought would have been a better fit, was *criminal. Your dad is a criminal.*

"I wish Mom would leave him," I said.

"I'm sure she'd be happier," Valerie said. I nodded to be agreeable, and in fact, I did agree, but I didn't want Valerie turning this into something about Mom's happiness. Mom was a woman who stayed with a man she knew might abuse her children.

Our conversation stalled. What other conversation was possible after that? The only thing we could do was agree that it was getting late, we should head home. I wanted her to tell me to come home with her. To live with her, Wayne, and the kids. Instead, we headed to the parking lot and got into our separate cars. As I was driving out of the parking lot, I saw Valerie driving toward me. She pulled up alongside me and rolled down her window. I rolled down mine.

"I'm so sorry that happened to you," she said. I told her that I'm sorry it happened to her, too.

I thought of Anna that night, and the odds that somehow, for some reason, Dad skipped Anna. Anna always said she didn't remember a thing about her childhood. But I knew that wasn't exactly true. Anna did have one memory.

Anna remembered being four. Mom and Dad were throwing a party and Anna got a new party dress just for the occasion. I imagined Anna dressed proudly, happy to be pretty and wanting nothing more than to show off to her daddy. She may have felt as if she was under the shadows of an outgoing sister and wanted — though her nature was to be reserved and quiet — to experience some of her sibling's glory. It would have taken a lot for Anna to go up to her father, seated at a table full of boisterous men, stop their conversation and say, "Look at my pretty new dress."

But she did. She stood by her dad, beaming, waiting for his approval, his kind words, and who knows, maybe even a warm fatherly embrace. What Anna got instead was a full bottle of beer poured over her head. Drenching her, and her new party dress, from head to toe. Dad laughed because it was a joke. Something like slapstick. The kind of thing you'd see in a Carry On gang movie. But no one at the party got the joke. Certainly not Anna.

I had heard that story and thought how I would willingly take on a hundred more encounters with my father — a thousand more abuses, public embarrassments, and shamings if that would spare Anna having beer poured on her new party dress. I would never forgive my dad for what he did to my sisters.

Our conversation plagued Valerie deeper than expected. But how could it not? Several weeks later she called me. She had talked to someone at her church who recommended that in cases such as this, it was best if things were kept quiet. Children aren't often believed in these situations, and it causes a rift in the family. And so, Valerie asked me to please not say anything. She said, "You might not be allowed back for Christmas, and I couldn't bear Christmas without you." She meant well. So, I agreed. But it did occur to me, why would it be me banned from Christmas and not my dad?

It would be years before Valerie and I spoke of it again.

I soon lost faith in the present and hope for the future, so long as it was clear to me that the past had all the answers. Too many secrets were left behind me, and there was only one person I knew who could reveal them all: I had to find the Wild Boy.

Chapter 20

On a summer's night in 1928, a local Waubamik farmer was shot while coming to the aid of John Burowski. What the farmer, Thomas Jackson, hadn't known was that Burowski and his accomplices had just robbed a train passing through Parry Sound. Burowski, or whoever had been driving the stolen getaway car, miscalculated a sharp bend in the road, sending the car careering into a nearby creek. When Burowski returned with Jackson, his associates had abandoned the vehicle and were never seen again. Oddly, they left the loot behind.

Friends of the owner of the stolen car, who had been tailing the bandits in a separate vehicle, confronted Burowski. Burowski drew a gun, a struggle ensued, shots were fired, and Jackson was killed. Despite the finding that the bullet had ricocheted off the car before hitting Jackson, Burowski was arrested, tried, and convicted of murder, then hanged in a Parry Sound jail. Nothing in Waubamik has since come close to matching the notoriety and the tragedy that came with Jackson's murder and Burowski's execution, unless you were a Fraser.

To find Waubamik you have to be looking, and even then it isn't guaranteed you won't drive by. Waubamik sits off Highway 124 between McDougall and McKellar, a brief drive outside of Parry Sound, northeast toward Sundridge. I'd been spending my summers working at a YMCA camp in Huntsville. Huntsville would be as close as I'd get to the Wild Boy as an adult.

That summer, I got all the information anyone could get off their birth certificate and a copy of their adoption papers. I knew I had been born at the Parry Sound General Hospital, but when I contacted the hospital, I was told there were no birth records dating back to 1958. They might have even said that the records burned in a fire, which would have been a wonderfully dramatic turn in the story and one I would have quickly morphed into my own little horror film scenario. Though maybe I had just been told that files were burned after a certain time had elapsed. But then this same person said that they knew the doctor who delivered all Parry Sound–area babies back then. *And he still lived in Parry Sound.*

I was told he was in the Parry Sound phone book.

The doctor answered the phone. I introduced myself, then told him when I was born, that I was adopted, and that he had likely delivered me. I said that he was the first contact — the first contact I had with the world and now my first contact with someone who had been there from the beginning. But the significance of it all seemed to be lost on the doctor, who waded through our conversation like it was a river stocked with sharks. There wasn't much hope that he'd remember delivering me, he said, not even if he had delivered all Parry Sound–area babies back then.

I knew from my birth certificate that the name I had been born with was Thomas John Fraser. I mentioned the Fraser name to the doctor. Yes, he knew my parents. And he knew that, although I had been born in the Parry Sound hospital, my home was in Waubamik.

Finding my biological parents became as easy as looking in the Parry Sound directory for a Fraser with a Waubamik address. There must have been only one Fraser in Waubamik, as I don't recall visiting more than one home. I arrived at the address certain that I found the right place. When no one answered my knock, I taped a message to the door.

A message was waiting for me when I got back to camp. If the Wild Boy had been forgotten, he was suddenly being remembered. It was just that no one expected he would show up taping notes to their front door. The home where I left the note was indeed occupied by a Fraser, but a cousin, not a parent. Her name was Bonnie, her message said, and she knew my parents — her Uncle Arnold and Aunt Dorothy. Both were alive and living in the same home where the Wild Boy had once played outside in the weeds and rocks and rubble.

I called Bonnie. We talked. She told me she had reached out to her aunt and uncle to let them know that their son had come back. Dorothy and Arnold, my birth parents, agreed to meet me. A week later, I returned to Waubamik, prepared to meet my parents and connect with the Wild Boy.

I met Bonnie at the house where I had left the note. Bonnie would be the first blood-related family member I met, a few years my senior, and yet able, so she claimed, to remember the Wild Boy. But her memories were vague, and I suspected they might be the product of stories passed down. "You're like a character from a book come to life," she said, and I realized that my sudden arrival was affecting more people than just Dorothy, Arnold, and me.

Bonnie directed me along the dirt-road tributaries branching off Highway 124. We'd have known each other for all of thirty minutes, discounting time spent on the phone, but we forwent talk about our own lives for a crash course in the history of Dorothy and Arnold Fraser.

I learned that the previous generation of Frasers had been explosive experts — with less emphasis on *expertise*, given that a great uncle is said to have blown himself up, Wile E. Coyote style, while blasting through Muskoka rock. And if the folklore is correct, then on that same day another uncle was killed during a hunting expedition.

Explosives-handling was not a trade Arnold got into. He thought himself a trapper, catching muskrat, beaver, and rabbit. From time to time he would take work with a road crew, just so long as it didn't require any skills beyond the use of a shovel and pick. But mostly Arnold did nothing. Dorothy was sweet, but sadly, next to Dorothy, Arnold looked like a genius. For good reason, though.

Bonnie tells me that "Dorothy's mother — your grandmother — played the piano, professionally. In concerts, I think, and there had been hopes for the same for Dorothy." But Bonnie explains that there had been an accident. At thirteen, Dorothy had been struck by a car, leaving her permanently brain damaged.

Bonnie wrapped up the history lesson with a story about me. But it really wasn't me at all. It was the Fraser kid, a wild boy who would stand outside with barely a stitch on, bruised, torn, and scabbed in all the usual places boys get bruised, torn, and scabbed, plus a few places that probably weren't usual. Bonnie says that all of Waubamik and some of Parry Sound knew the boy. They'd see him playing, or playing the best anyone could in a sunbaked lot filled with tin cans and rusty car parts. And with him always was his only toy: a headless doll. That kid and his doll were a bit of a local fixture.

There was a pause and then Bonnie reiterated, as though it could be forgotten, the extent of Dorothy and Arnold's poverty and their lack of education. "Neither of them are too bright," she said. "Prepare yourself for a shock. They don't have much in the way of anything."

She said this several times during the drive, as though it could not be said often enough. It occurred to me that Bonnie's warning had less to do with preparing me for what was ahead, than it did with protecting her aunt and uncle. I sensed from her an apprehension, as though she suddenly feared she was leading the hunter to the hunted. How awful it would be to bring her aunt and uncle their lost son, if it meant having them witness his disgust and disappointment?

I promised Bonnie to put my expectations on hold.

We drove along dirt roads, past shambles of forgotten houses and tumbled barns. This was the scenic route on the way to the Frasers. Eventually, we pulled into a lot scattered with scraps of metal in various stages of being reclaimed by forest weeds.

But there was no house, only an abandoned delivery truck, anchored on cinder blocks, pushed up against the side of what might be called a shed. The shed had all the structure and soundness of a child's backyard fort. There were mismatched planks tacked along the walls, and thick sheets of plastic nailed over spots of exposed pink insulation. And everywhere cats scavenging the ruins like a horde of rodents.

Bonnie had me park the car in front of the shed. Other than the broken-down truck, there were no other vehicles.

"Here we are," she said. A hint of defiance in her voice dared me to be critical. A take-it-or-leave-it proclamation. She looked past me, indicating with a glance that the shed was indeed the house. I felt if I were to express any reaction, shock, amazement, or pity, Bonnie would turn the car around and drive me back. We left the car, walked toward the house through the minefield of cats who cowered but refused to relinquish their ground. A metal screen door hung on rusty hinges. Bonnie called out a "Hello," opened the screen door, and walked in without the courtesy of a knock.

Three people waited inside. The room had the look of an early settler's homestead, but one that had been abandoned and then reclaimed by squatters. The first person I saw — the only one of the three who was standing — was Dorothy. My mother.

Dorothy stood by the doorway, poised like the centrepiece in a Shelby Lee Adams photograph, an Appalachian figure caught by the camera in a moment of surprise and confusion. She was shorter than me. Skinny on top but wider and fuller in the waist and in the hips. Her hair was dark — is it possible she dyed it? — capped with a pronounced cowlick that hovered above her forehead like a question mark. She stared at me through dark-rimmed glasses, then reached out to embrace me. I allowed it. What it must have meant for her to hold her child, now fully grown. To be with the child for the first time in almost twenty years. A child she had no reason to believe that she would see again. I imagined her taking me in with her breath, her sight, and her touch, absorbing all that I was to fill the empty space between her last memory of me and the me that stood before her. Behind her two men sat at a table pushed into a corner. The older man I knew would be Arnold — my father. Arnold looked up from his chair with the same cursory interest one client gives another when walking into a barbershop. I read his reaction as disinterest, but it might have been an inability to grasp how the past could so easily catch up to him. He gave Dorothy her time with me. Was she looking for something left in me for her to remember, something in my eyes, my face, something to feel beneath her fingers when she touched me?

Sitting at the table with Arnold was a young man, handsome, I thought, if it weren't for the bone-deep grime covering his face and hands. I hadn't expected a third person to be invited to this mother-and-child reunion. I might have been offended, had I not noticed the remarkable resemblance he had to the Wild Boy. And the kicker? His name was Tommy. My namesake, Dorothy told me.

Tommy stood up to greet me. I hadn't expected him to rise, neither did I expect him to smile, but he did. He was disarmingly pleasant, somewhat bashful, and polite. He held out his hand for me to shake. In that moment I understood how I must look to others. I shook Tommy's hand wondering if he, too, were taken aback by our resemblance.

I wasn't quite able to follow Dorothy's convoluted family trail that led to Tommy's existence and why he was here, but I was left with the impression that he was a distant cousin. I don't know what I was expecting, not a brother — Bonnie would have said something — but a cousin didn't make much sense.

As for the mail truck, it was not as abandoned as I had thought. That was where Tommy slept. So, it would seem I had been replaced. There was a strange comfort in knowing they weren't entirely capable of life without me, and that the Wild Boy had his chance to live and grow in a world that was intended to be mine. But Tommy — my distant cousin? How did he feel now that the original had returned? Was he ever able to *be*, or had he always lived as a filler in someone else's life?

My attention turned away from Tommy and back to Dorothy and Arnold. I wanted to see them not as strangers but as people I instinctively recognized; an inherent familiarity drawing me to them, as if being there was migratory; an inescapable pull or calling. Perhaps it had been, even if I couldn't feel it then.

Their poverty was significant, but Dorothy and Arnold (and Tommy) took to their surroundings with unapologetic ease, comfortable with what they had, equally comfortable with what they didn't. I had never been wealthy, but this was foreign enough that I was able to romanticize it as a history that might have been mine. This would have been my home. The delivery truck my room, decorated how? With car parts? Posters of heavy metal bands? Calendar girls? How different would I have been?

The reunion was a one-way street and not the tender nor dramatic scenario written in books or re-enacted in movies. I would romanticize it later, to friends and family, but for the time being it was a reunion based on biology, and curiosity, a selfish visit to take what I wanted with no thought of leaving anything behind. We were strangers, no matter how hard Dorothy and Arnold (mostly Dorothy) revived memories of the Wild Boy they would take camping along the trap lines, the kid who played in the dirt out front, and in the dirt inside or whose favourite toy was a headless doll. She told me of having lost control of the baby carriage with me inside, laughing as it careered to the bottom of a hill. Not a banner example of good parenting, but I did like the image of me as fearless and hoped that the story was true.

"You tried to pat a massasauga rattler. But I got to you in time. Not that it mattered, that snake was more afraid of you than you were of it." I felt a stronger connection when she told me of a younger sister named Rose. She said I wouldn't know about her because Rose was born after I left. I was curious about her use of the word *left*, as though I had abandoned her. Dorothy's eyes never left me, as though fearful I would disappear again. I knew this because I was able to look away. It was a struggle to see where I was in her eyes and face. But the only resemblance was the cowlick. I wish I knew what Dorothy saw when she looked at me. Did she see the man she had found or the child she had lost?

Arnold lifted himself up from his chair. He was a bear of a man, with eyes shrouded beneath heavy lids. A mountain man without a mountain. On his head was a shock of hair jutting out in tousled spires of grey. His pants were hefted up by suspenders over a sizable belly, a red flannel shirt tucked half in with the other half of the shirt caught in the grip of the suspenders, draping over his waistband like a handkerchief carelessly stuffed in a pocket. I expected him to shake my hand, slap me on the back, sucker-punch me in the shoulder, but he opened his arms as though coming in for a hug, which was exactly what he was doing. The bristles from his unshaven face scratched my cheek but the hug was gratifying, and not the uncomfortable awkwardness I expected. It didn't matter that I was getting a hug from a stranger; what mattered was that this man was giving a hug to a son he remembered. It was not lost on me that this was an embrace that expected nothing in return.

"How is Violet?" he asked.

I didn't know who he meant.

"Your sister," Dorothy said, as though the fault in memory was mine. "We were told that they kept you together." But I didn't know of Violet and had only just learned of Rose. For me it was a thrill to discover two previously unknown younger sisters, but it was cold comfort to Dorothy, who believed her children had always had each other.

I could sense Bonnie's discomfort at not wanting to be witness to her aunt's and uncle's sadness. Tommy must have blended into the mosaic of mismatched bits of furniture and the scattered pages from fishing and hunting magazines and old calendars, for I don't remember seeing him anymore.

But if Dorothy was at all pained by this, she didn't let it show. She simply carried on with stories of my past, rhyming them off like shared memories and not just her own. Only now these memories also included a little girl named Violet.

I can piece together a somewhat fantastical and occasionally contradictory history of my birth parents, Dorothy and Arnold, plus something of their life with the Wild Boy.

Most of the stories I heard came from Dorothy and Arnold on the ride back to Bonnie's place. Bonnie had arranged a reunion of sorts — a gathering of about fifteen people, mostly Arnold's half-siblings and their children — in honour of my unexpected return.

Bonnie rode back with Tommy while Dorothy and Arnold rode with me, choosing to sit in the back seat.

I heard of Arnold's mishaps with the law; how he missed the bend at the end of Highway 126 and drove straight into the lake (for the second time in three years), drowning the car in eight feet of water, the tires sinking a foot deeper into a murky bottom of algae and slime, and Arnold crawling out of the car and onto the shore more sober than he was going in. Arnold ended the story with "I own a used car lot — it's just off of Highway 126 at the bottom of the lake."

People loved hearing Arnold's stories (according to Arnold), especially the McKinnon girls, daughters of his half-sister, May, who'd affectionately dubbed him their "Uncle Barney with the goo-goo-googly eyes" after a silly little song their mother sang.

Dorothy's stories weren't as funny.

Not much of anything had been expected of Dorothy since the accident, least of all any hope for life as a concert pianist. And so, when she met, then married, her first husband, an indecent man with a decent job working on the northern highway road crew, there was no reason for her to believe that things weren't right on track.

"They aren't breaking down the door," her mother had said.

Arnold didn't like Dorothy's first husband but tolerated him because he was his crew's foreman. Arnold, when sober enough to know which end of the shovel to hold, needed the work.

"He wasn't nice to your mom," said Arnold. "Called her stupid. I never thought there was anything wrong with Dorothy. She looked smart. She wore glasses, for God's sake." Arnold told me that he and Dorothy saw each other only when the road crew got together to drink, which I suppose was often enough. One night Dorothy's husband picked up a bottle of Canadian whisky and, in a generous moment, shared the bottle with the crew. Dorothy jumped in to remind Arnold that he hadn't been invited, he had just tagged along.

Arnold continued with his story: "He was saying that she was too stupid to tie her own shoes, which made us look at her shoes to see if that were true, and yep, sure enough, laces undone. She just looked at her feet and started laughing."

Dorothy and Arnold started to spend more time together, and since no one messes with a Fraser, not many questions were asked. And when the road crew finished up that year and moved to the next town, Dorothy stayed behind. Not that her husband took any notice. Didn't even bother to get a divorce.

"I don't think he knew Dorothy was pregnant when he left," said Arnold.

And that is how I learned that I was not her only child; indeed, I wasn't even her first child. My sister Elsie was born two years before my arrival. And, according to Bonnie, this was when Dorothy and Arnold's world filled with happiness. And, to the extent that Dorothy and Arnold could comprehend the moods of others, it was a time when the world was happiest for them.

It wouldn't last.

Chapter 21

- - - - - - - - - - -

What Dorothy recalled about the day of the fire on November 5, 1957, was how cold it was in the morning. Cold enough that her nostrils pinched shut and her lungs would prickle from breathing in the frigid air.

"Too cold to get out of bed," she said, and so she remained beneath the weight of the blankets, heavy and warm. In another room, she could hear her nieces as they squabbled through their morning routine of frustrations and short-term annoyances.

"During the colder months we would stay with Arnold's half-sister, May," Dorothy explained.

In Dorothy's version of the fire, Arnold began the morning wheezing, farting, and coughing — an inharmonious orchestra of waking sounds. If Arnold was affected by the cold, it came second to the urge for a smoke. He sat on the edge of the bed, clawing for the pack of cigarettes left balancing overnight on the windowsill. Dorothy hauled the blankets over her shoulders.

"It felt like the end of the world," she told me, managing to squeeze humour in a story that was building toward the worst day of her life.

Arnold lit the cigarette, pulled on a pair of pants he had dropped to the floor, and left the room.

It was here that Dorothy interjected her own story with a strange plea as though she were delivering a public service announcement. "You have to tell your father to quit smoking," she said. "You know he only listens to you." Dorothy was erasing years of exile, recreating a life imagined and positioning my return as a routine —'nothing more than a visit from her adult son. I didn't try to correct her. I allowed the comment to pass unchallenged, then pressed her to continue the story.

She described hearing Elsie's voice coming from the other room; the bah and coos and raspberries of a toddler. Elsie slept with her cousins in their crammed room of box springs and mattresses and errant pieces of board games and doll clothes. Then there was May's voice asking Florence, the eldest of her girls, my cousins, to fetch the can of kerosene from out back.

Arnold came back into the bedroom, the cigarette dangling from his mouth. He was holding Elsie, who was wide awake and beaming on the promise of a new day. Dorothy smiled at her baby: a bundle wrapped in sweater over sweater over sweater. Her rosy cheeks waved precariously close to the amber glow that burned at the end of Arnold's cigarette.

"I warned Arnold, be careful. Don't you burn her," Dorothy said.

So, Arnold passed Elsie off to Dorothy, but Elsie inched her way from Dorothy's arms and lowered herself onto the floor where she found something in a pile of clothes to amuse her.

Arnold went back into the other room.

In the other room, May was bent over a wood-burning stove, piling chunks of wood into the small cast-iron opening.

Arnold announced that he was going into town.

The front door opened. Florence entered, her pace slowed by the weight of a red can of kerosene. She tugged it inside, both hands gripping the handle, the sound of the liquid sloshing against the inside walls of the container. She struggled with her load from the front door to the wood stove. The front door remained open.

Florence put the kerosene in front of her mother then returned to close the front door. And that's where Dorothy remembered Florence standing when the fire started. May splashed the kerosene onto the logs and the empty cereal packages.

I was left to imagine much of the rest; how the kerosene fumes would have risen like aroma lines coming off an apple pie in a comic strip. How the room would have filled with the acrid smell of kerosene, singeing their breath with a forewarning that none of them read. I imagined Arnold with a cigarette still burning between his fingers watching as May put match to chemical.

In my version of the fire, I hear Arnold say, "That ought to get 'er going."

Dorothy remembered Elsie calling from the bedroom, a toddler's frustration at being left alone.

And so, May would have struck the match against the sandpaper edge of a matchbox once, then again and then a third time before the phosphorous end spit and sparked in dancing hues of yellow and orange before settling into a single flame. She'd have touched flame to the wood drunk on kerosene. But instead of a satisfying whoosh of flames engulfing wood, there was something else; the sound of a baseball bat hitting the side of the stove. Flames would have shot over the edge of the stove, then just as quickly receded; the adults falling back shielding themselves from the heat with their forearms. May toppled to the floor, Arnold slammed into the coffee table, falling ass-over-teakettle onto the ashtrays and beer cans that were scattered on top.

Dorothy said it reminded her of a Bible story: Shadrach, Meshach, and Abednego, standing unharmed in the fiery furnace.

The fire would send kernels of sparks jumping from the stove's open grate. Flames furled around the cast-iron frame. The intensity of the heat would have driven them farther from the stove.

I imagine a trail of kerosene spilling onto the cement podium where the stove stood. At first, the drops would pool harmlessly on the concrete until enough flames gathered to create a fiery stream that trickled toward the edge. Tiny embers would drop onto the floor, disappearing in tiny bursts no more harmful than soap bubbles. But when the embers disappeared beneath cracks in the floor, where old newspapers and sawdust insulated the space between the living room and the rock base beneath the house, where the dry November leaves had blown and rested alongside paper debris and forgotten toys, the fire quietly snaked a route below the house, rising again through the floorboards, finding first the couch and then the curtains before climbing up the wallpapered walls in a rush of flames worthy of a Vegas magician making a spectacular entrance.

Dorothy's next memory is of Elsie. Where was Elsie? Elsie was still in the bedroom. But the flames, which had now engulfed the curtains, curled along the wallpaper, and left the couch smoldering, had reached the bedroom door frame. Dorothy remembers the doorknob burning her hand, but she didn't let go. She pushed open the door, thinking only about getting to her child and not how the closed door would have been a divider between the child and the smoke and flames. Dorothy believes she caught a glimpse of her daughter still sitting by the pile of clothes. There was no sound other than the violent snap of wood panels being torn apart by flame, curling up at the corners and turning black before the open door flooded the bedroom with fire and turned it into an inescapable furnace.

My cousins ran from the house. The three adults stayed to fight the blaze long after they knew it was too late to save Elsie. May might have been the first to understand this and pulled Dorothy away from the burning room and into the open air where the two women collapsed, the fresh air pushing in on their smoke-filled lungs.

Arnold only remembers getting out of the house, running to the back with an axe and hacking at the outside wall. The girls cried while watching their Uncle Barney with the goo-goo-googly eyes smash the blade of the axe against layers of insulation and wood, desperate to break down the wall and free his child.

Two days later an article appeared in the local paper. The story and headline read:

Two-Year-Old Dies in Early Morning Fire

Elsie May Fraser, aged 2, was burned to death when the home of Mr. and Mrs. Joseph McKinnon was destroyed by fire in Waubamik on Wednesday, November 5. The fire started at 6:30 a.m. when Mrs. McKinnon attempted to light a wood stove, using kerosene. In the hospital are Mr. and Mrs. Fraser and Mrs. McKinnon, who were severely burned before escaping from the building. The three children of the McKinnons', Florence, 9, Maxine, 7, and Viola, 6, were taken out unharmed.

Mr. McKinnon was not home at the time of the fire.

Mr. Fraser received cuts as he attempted to chop a hole in the side of the house to rescue his baby. As the air reached the heated interior, it burst into flames.

Drs. Malkin and Howes attended the injured people in hospital. Dr. A.J.L. Wright, Coroner, and Corporal Howard Gunn, of the local OPP investigated.

Right below the article, in the same column, is the headline, in block letters:

FIFTIETH WEDDING ANNIVERSARY

A gaily decorated Legion Hall in Magnetawan was the setting for a dinner party given by the family of Mr. and Mrs. Lewis Crossman to celebrate their 50th wedding anniversary.

There it was, the death of a two-year-old girl flowing gracefully into the notice of a fifty-year wedding celebration.

Five months after the fire, in the middle of his mother's worst nightmare, the Wild Boy was born: a howling, screaming intrusion on the memory of his mother's lost child.

Several years later, not long after meeting Dorothy and Arnold, I found Viola, one of the cousins who survived the fire, now an accountant living in London, Ontario. Viola told me that she didn't remember anything about the fire, only that it happened and that she was there. And no, I cannot call May. May, her mother, my aunt, never forgave herself for not knowing that you don't use kerosene to light an indoor fire.

Viola was curious about me, though. She wondered if I looked at all like my father, the uncle she adored. The one with the goo-goo-googly eyes.

Chapter 22

I've seen only two photographs from the Frasers. One is of Elsie, that I assume was taken not long before her death, although when a child dies at two, any photograph taken is a photograph taken not long before death. But what did I know of pictures and babies? She may have been a hardy, healthy one-year-old when that photo was snapped with a solid year still ahead of her.

The photograph was black-and-white, with the white glossy border familiar in photos of a certain era. I wondered who took it, who had owned the camera, who took the film in to be developed, who paid for all of this so that it could eventually end up in my parents' hands.

In the photo Elsie wears a dress, white and clean. It flows from her in perfect little-girl frills, like she was dressed for church or someone's wedding. Perhaps she was. There is no one left to ask. On her face is a light scowl that makes her look impatient rather than unhappy, as if too much play time has been swallowed up by posing for this picture. In the picture she's sitting on a rock as big as a boulder. The landscape around her looks barren. No grass, mostly rocks and weeds, an abandoned lot in the middle of nowhere. A rural ghetto. Elsie sits in front of a house: a one-level, rectangular-shaped, wood-framed house lifted on a bed of cinder blocks. Was this the McKinnon house where Elsie died?

The other photo is a picture of me. It, too, is in black-and-white. I put my age at about four months old in this photograph, given the pudginess of my features. I'm seen from waist up, shirtless, sitting up in a baby carriage, my hair not fully grown in but cropped to my scalp as though it were painted on. In my hand I clutch a headless doll; my face is turned to the camera. I stare directly at the photographer, with an expression that seems to be saying, *Hey, what the hell is that? A camera? How is it we can afford a camera when my doll doesn't even have head?*

Looking at the picture now, I assume the photograph was taken with the same camera that took the photo of Elsie. I also assume the carriage and the headless doll were once Elsie's, too. A couple of thoughts occur to me. One, that my parents didn't wait a year or so before taking my picture — just in case — and two, that, even though they were likely lost in inconsolable grief, they still thought enough to give me a toy, even if it was a headless doll that might have belonged to my dead sister.

These would have been the days I spent muddying through the puddles of rain that collect in the crevices and the dips of an otherwise rocky and hardened terrain, happily ignorant of the poverty and neglect that others feared would threaten my future.

I'm told that I was walking by the time Violet, my new sister, was born. I had developed a premature sense for nurturing so much so that it was me, rather than our parents, who was first to attend to Violet when she cried. I was a pint-sized caregiver stumbling toward a crib that several months earlier had been mine. I doted on my little sister like I was her sole provider, happy, I suppose, to have had something other than a headless doll to play with.

If there are photos of Violet, I have not seen them. But I do know that for Dorothy and Arnold, Violet was a blessing. She was the rebirth of Elsie, a blue-eyed little girl for them to cherish. Their second chance at happiness. So, when Children's Aid took Violet away, they must have felt that their happiness had left, and I must have felt the absence of someone to care for.

A few days later *they* came back for me. My time with the Frasers came to an end. None of the memories of the three years I spent as a Fraser remain.

But I have a reoccurring dream. In it I am playing in a yard full of rocks and weeds, behind me is a house. A car pulls up. It's a dark sedan, shiny, seemingly unscathed by the dust and gravel that would have sprayed up as it drove along the dirt road. The car door opens. A man steps out, perhaps two, and walks over to a little girl not far from me. The man picks up the little girl and takes her into the car, the door shuts. In a moment, a woman steps out of the house. Thinking back on the dream, the woman could be Dorothy. The woman yells as the car pulls away, not screaming, but frantic. I can't make out what she says. And then, the woman (Dorothy?) looks down at me and says, "You were supposed to look after her."

Of course, the Children's Aid don't kidnap little girls playing in front of their parent's home. Of course, mothers don't leave three-year-olds to look after their infant siblings. But in dreams, weird things can happen.

Chapter 23

- - - - - - - - -

There was no shortage of people to explain to me how lucky I was.

"Well, well, well …" they said, "you're going to get your own mommy and daddy. Aren't you the lucky one?"

And I could only answer "Yes, I am," because when a grown-up tells you that you're one of the lucky ones, then you have no choice but to believe them, even if you don't know why it is that you're so lucky.

My good fortune included not only a new mommy and daddy, but a home on Royal Street in a town called Waterloo. I imagined Waterloo to be a very dangerous place filled with rivers and lakes and ponds and streams. My memory of that day has been idealized over the years. I was three pushing four.

The woman who drove me to my new home said she doesn't recall there being any lakes and rivers in Waterloo, but we'd just have to wait and see. Still, I worried no one thought to pack rainboots.

"You're looking quite sharp with your brand new clothes and haircut," she said, then she crinkled her nose like a rabbit downwind of a carrot patch. "I think someone has Brylcreem in their hair."

My hand touched the slick strands of hair brushed into place
and held tight by whatever ointment was massaged onto my scalp,
an ointment that filled the car with the heavy scent of too many
flowers blossoming at once. My hand became coated in an oily
film that I immediately wiped on my new crayon-sun-yellow shirt.
It was my first button-down shirt, and the first shirt with a collar
that's been folded like the wings on a paper airplane. New pants,
too: short, blue, and sturdy as drapes.

"Now, let's keep an eye out for a sign that says Royal Street. Do
you know what *Royal* means?"

I did, thanks to a recent run of picture books depicting handsome princes, and sleeping princesses, regal queens, and roly-poly,
red-cheeked kings.

"Rich people who live in castles."

This made her laugh, which was all I needed to want to stay
with her forever.

"Well, I suppose that's true. But it also means kings and queens,
and princes and princesses. You're going to live on a street named
for royalty. Isn't that something?"

"And dragons," I added, because the best thing about story
books with kings and queens in them are the dragons.

"No, I don't think there are any dragons."

But I can tell she's not sure. Just because you don't see the dragons doesn't mean there are no dragons.

"Why? Do you like dragons? I would think dragons would be
scary."

"Oh, yes." I had the confidence of a child experienced in the ways
of dragons. "Dragons are scary. But I know how to fight them."

The woman filled our travel time with stories about what it
would be like to have a mom and dad. I hadn't given much thought
to having my own mom and dad. Why would I? Whenever I needed
a grown-up, and even times when I didn't, one was always there

picking me up, putting me down, feeding me, dressing me, annoying me. Moms and dads were everywhere. It hadn't occurred to me that you can have a pair of your own.

"You're my mommy," I said, as if the decision were mine. I'd grown attached to this woman, just as I had grown attached to the several women who rushed through my life before her. Falling in love was easy, a life skill I carried with me to varying degrees of success and failure. But then my prerequisite for love was based solely on kindness. It is a simple equation: kindness becomes beauty and beauty becomes love. I remember this woman sitting beside me, the way her dark hair stopped at her shoulders, the blue dress she wore, and the scarf around her neck held together by a silver clasp with the tips of that scarf jutting out like rabbit ears. She was the picture perfect mom cut straight from a magazine ad that depicts a young family caught in a moment of joy as they drive off in their new 1962 Cadillac.

"Oh, sweetheart, I can't be your mommy. I'm already a mommy to someone else. You have your own mommy, and she's waiting for us, right now. You'll see. We'll be there soon. Okay?"

"Okay," I said, or at least I said something close to it. Something agreeable. I didn't argue or plead or whine. I had no reason. Not that I could be specific about it, but I understood how these things happen. I'd developed a sense of people coming and going without warning. And whenever one person left, someone new stepped in. This was nothing new; still, if I was to have a mommy, then this woman driving seemed perfectly fit for the job.

The woman smiled at me. I thought perhaps she'd changed her mind, but her smile was just as she told me that I was the handsomest little boy she'd ever seen. Those words filled me with an unknown joy. To be handsome must be a wonderful thing. I decided that I would be handsome forever. And as much as possible, I've remained true to that decision.

"Oh, there's a sign over there. What do you think it says?"

I looked to where she pointed and indeed there was a sign, although, without the ability to read, I could only assume that it said something wonderful, like *Warning! Dragons Ahead.*

"Do you think it says Royal Street?"

Okay. Yeah. Probably.

I nodded.

"I think so, too. Let's give it a try, shall we?"

If this wasn't Royal Street, then we were heading toward nowhere without hope of turning back. The idea was not entirely bad. If we kept driving past Waterloo, through the puddles and the lakes, past the castles and palaces on Royal Street, drove until there was no more road to drive on, then the two of us could just sit there at the end of the road and marvel at how far we had come.

If the decision were mine.

The dark-haired woman rolled down the car window, allowing a spring breeze to carry in the smells and sounds of a Saturday unique to a Saturday on Royal Street. I stayed seated for this part of the trip, stretching my neck to peer out the side window looking for signs of castles and kings and dragons and palaces. There were only rows of houses, one after another, lined on both sides of the road. Too many to count. A sidewalk stretched the length of the street, then curved where the street ended and continued down the next. Young maple trees that were too narrow and weak to climb spotted the manicured lawns, their leaves clenched inside tiny sprouts not yet ready to face the cool April air. Flower boxes hung on windowsills, empty but for the fresh mound of store-bought earth churned up inside. Tiny mounds of dirt appeared beneath bay windows and alongside driveways, waiting to be tended to with plants and flowers. Neatly sculpted shrubs added a lasting green outside the homes and along the footpaths that led to the front doors.

"I think I see your new home. We certainly did a fine job of finding our way, didn't we? You're a great little navigator."

"Yeah," I said proudly, not knowing anything about navigators but happy to know that I was a good one.

The house was a brown bungalow. It was a house unlike any I had seen before, not a palace, not a castle as I had hoped, but still one of the nicest homes I had ever seen, new enough to look as if untouched by rain or snow; a house that sprouted up from the ground as naturally and perfectly as the maple tree in the front yard.

The woman slowed down and turned the car onto the driveway. "There they are," she said. Three people stood smiling in the frame of the entranceway as if wary of stepping out any farther.

The woman shifted the car into park and turned off the engine. It was then with the sudden silence of the car and the stillness after being in constant motion, that my world stopped. I shrank back into my seat, burying myself into the upholstery. The people in the doorway kept smiling. Maybe they wouldn't want me and the woman driving would have no choice but to be my mother.

The woman, who couldn't be my mother because she was already the mother of someone else, turned to me and smiled. "Come," she said. "Let's meet your new family." ·

I didn't move until the woman walked to the passenger side, opened the door, and coaxed me out of the car. "It's going to be wonderful," she said. And she took my hand and lead me inside to begin my new life.

Chapter 24

- - - - - - - - - - - -

His Alzheimer's came on slowly, spreading over him with a childlike gentleness; the innocence he overtook now overtaking him. Mom and Dad had moved into a granny flat my sister Anna and her husband, James, had put up on their lot. Mom often said, in jest and in anger, that one day she was going to run away and live in the bush. It seemed she had gotten her wish. James had built a dream home for Anna on a massive acreage of forest filled with undergrowth, wildlife, a spring-fed stream. But the reality of living in the bush, isolated with a man who increasingly became a stranger, was not as idyllic as Mom imagined. She cried the day they left the house in Kitchener and moved into the granny flat.

Mom noticed the forgetfulness: objects he could no longer name, friends he no longer recognized. He started wetting the bed. And then one January morning, after months of his leaving kettles boiling atop of burners and wandering the bush looking for his brother, Quinnie, long dead and buried, Mom looked out the window of the granny flat and saw Dad on the snow-covered lawn with a leaf rake, raking leaves.

I missed much of my dad's descent into his disease. I had been living in Toronto for twenty-plus years, floundering above poverty level, occasionally dipping below, living off romance and surviving on the kindness of girlfriends, taking advantage of their ski chalets and cottages. Getting high, then gorging on food and drink, adding to an ongoing tab at exclusive sports clubs where their parents were members — places where the Wild Boy was not allowed to go. I had become, it would seem, something of a con man, managing privilege with naive charm and a youthful aspiration to become a writer. *The Talented Mr. Ripley* with a North American backdrop. Eventually the charm fizzled into disappointment and the women who loved me (and whom I ineffectively loved in return) would shake their heads as if waking from under a spell and take their leaves. The Wild Boy laughed and said he always knew when a relationship ended because he could hear the weight fall from the girl's parents' shoulders.

After decades of therapy, I landed a dream job with a public broadcaster in Toronto: a movie show hosted by an amiable man named Elwy Yost. Dad would have been impressed. The Wild Boy had all but left, appearing only occasionally, late at night, or catching me off guard when I was in places I was unsure that I belonged.

I rarely found reason to return home, but on one occasion my friend Bruce was driving back to Kitchener for a poker game with a group of friends from university. We drove down together and crashed for the night at a friend's house after the game, waking up with hash-and-booze hangovers. I needed to be back in Toronto that night for a date with a woman I'd seen only in a photograph on a colleague's desk. I only knew that her name was Nicole. But before heading back, I convinced Bruce to drive by my parents' home. It was spring. There was a chill, but it was sunny. The sprouting leaves and plants in bloom made the country drive enjoyable.

We found the house; the branches and foliage of the trees were still sparse enough that the house could be seen from the road.

Bruce turned into the lane that wound down a hill. Mom's granny flat was at the bottom of the hill. Bruce parked. The lane continued on toward the larger house with a parking pad large enough for four cars. Garden boxes ran neatly along the front of the flat.

My mom's home resembled a parked trailer covered in wood panelling; a small summer cottage kept neat and bright by an elderly couple who had nothing to do but keep their home in prime condition.

Curiosity brought Mom to the side window — visitors were rare. Bruce and I stepped out of the car. So did the Wild Boy. Mom wouldn't have recognized Bruce's car, and probably not Bruce, but me she recognized and came to the back door of the flat to let us in.

"Thom, what a nice surprise," she said, leading Bruce and me into the kitchen/living/dining room. Dad was wearing his blue suit, the jacket off, but the vest on and a tie secured nicely into a Windsor knot. Dad had dressed for church, even though they no longer went.

"Every day he does this," Mom explained. "He shines the shoes, picks out a clean dress shirt, ties his tie, puts on his suit, and waits all day for church to start." Dad had become so devoted a fan of the scriptures that even God would have found him extreme, but would, no doubt, still be impressed with his ability to tie a Windsor knot.

Dad leaned on the counter of the galley kitchen, led there by Mom. She tended to him the way a mother would tend to a toddler. Dad grinned at Bruce and me. Grinning seemed to be the only means of communication he had left.

"Look who's here, Clare," Mom said, making sure he was looking in my direction and not Bruce's.

She then moved his attention toward Bruce. "And you remember his friend Bruce." He didn't. I could sense his confusion. We all did. Bruce stood with me in the space that made up their living area, wishing, I presumed, that he had declined the suggestion to drop by.

There was not much in way of conversation. We spoke in short, polite, and forgettable sentences. We weren't invited to sit down, and neither did they sit.

Dad stared at us, his eyes vacant, as though attempting to determine which one of us, Bruce or me, was his son. Assuming he knew he had a son. He looked, as Wayne recently described, like a "sweet old man." But I still knew who he was. I tried to find sympathy. It would have been the right reaction, and Mom would have been comforted had I shown sadness or concern, but the Wild Boy wouldn't allow it. The Wild Boy saw his innocence and sweetness as a cruel mask covering his true self.

You know where I've seen those vacant eyes and Cheshire grin before? the Wild Boy asked. *They remind me of you — your vacant eyes and Cheshire grin, years back when you were locked in shock, shame, and confusion. Whenever you had to leave your body.*

No, I couldn't find the sympathy I needed, but there was regret. Not because I was unable to forgive, but because I knew that I had let him get away with it. He was gone. He'd become harmless. Unable to recall names, unable to know what time church starts, unable to harm children.

It was the last time I'd see Dad alive.

Chapter 25

B y the time Nicole meets my dad, he's already dead. To every casket there is a silk lining, and on that lining lay the newly deceased, tucked in like a newborn. His shoulders squared, face forward, hands folded on his chest, dressed forever in the blue pinstripe suit that he had worn for years to every significant event, none more significant than this. Dad looks worn and ready for rest, but the suit, the suit looks new. And not just a clean-and-measured-and-tapered-to-fit-the-corpse new, but fresh-off-the-rack-ready-to-wear new. That's because Dad took diligent care of the things he loved. He was meticulous in the care he gave to car, home, and personal appearance. He regularly washed the dust and road salt from the car, he dug the weeds out of the lawn and raked it clear of fallen leaves, he trimmed the grass to a uniform length that would rival the level bristles on a sea cadet's crewcut, he shovelled snow from the walk and driveway so that nothing but the asphalt showed through, his shoes were polished to a military sheen, and his clothes were ironed, hung up, or folded as need be.

Moments earlier Nicole and I had pulled into the gravelled parking lot of the Velvet Hills Baptist Church, a single-storey, unadorned concrete house of worship nestled in a vacant field not far off from the sideroad that leads into Heidelberg. This was my parents' church, a Christian warehouse for the charismatic and the faithful, a place for believers to cleanse their souls and give praise to their Lord. "Victoria," the name Nicole gave to the voice of our Garmin GPS that we stuck to the front windshield like a second rear-view mirror, talked us along Highway 8 through Kitchener and past Waterloo until we hit Wagner's Corners, over-enunciating each letter and syllable of the street names and numbers with robotic precision. "In Five. HunDred. MeTers turn left at WagOnErs. CorNers." But, as delightful as she might sound, I'd have found my way to Velvet Hills without Victoria's help, having been here before in my own fruitless search for redemption.

We walk into the open foyer of the church where family members and friends, many of whom I no longer recognize or remember, mill about in groups engaging in polite exchanges. Someone's laugher flows through the foyer like tinkling glass. And then there is a silence when someone notices us entering the room.

Being the only son of the deceased makes one's entrance notable. A few of the mourners don't know who I am, given that I've been distant from my father for many years, but they quickly learn through the whispers and explanation from others. The acoustics of the foyers allows me to hear them despite their lowered voices. I'm not bothered by what they say.

That's Clare's son.

His son? I didn't know he had a son.

He's adopted. They never got along. I'm surprised he came.

And for others, a different fascination takes hold. I am a face they've seen on television as host of a well-known movie show. Either way, the weight of their attention sits well with me. Nicole feels it, too.

"This is not about you," Nicole whispers to me, not to be unkind but to ground me in the moment before my ego takes over and I start greeting people as though they were gathered to see me.

"I think it's a little bit about me," I reply in an answer that sounds more hopeful than certain.

Nicole takes my hand and leads us toward Mom, who stands with my sisters and their husbands. Mom seems, at least for now, to be in control of her emotions. Has she put her mourning behind her? Her face reveals nothing but the dominance of a lone matriarch. *Is it possible that she's angry that I showed up?*

"Good," Mom says, keeping her hands folded in front of her, "I'm glad you could make it."

"Of course I made it." I fear I'm being too confrontational. Nicole squeezes my hand to pull me back in. Mom turns her head toward the casket, dismissing me, so I can pay respects to the deceased. People step aside, making room for us to approach the casket. I feel them studying our faces, looking for hints of emotion and signs of our loss. It must seem to them that I am a cold and unremorseful son. I find it hard to feign sorrow. Even harder to feign respect.

Dad's expressionless face, now heavily caked in a powdery skintone base, looks to me not like that of a man "peacefully at rest," as is said of the recently deceased, but like the face of a man entombed in a motionless body, holding back painful secrets behind closed eyes. *But what does it matter, if there is no heaven or hell? No reward and no punishment?*

"So," I whisper to Nicole, taking her closer to my father's body, "there he is." I say this as if presenting a long-awaited project that's finally complete. *Voila!* is on the tip of my tongue, but I think better of it.

"Do you not think it's odd that the first time I meet your father is at his funeral?" she asks.

"Maybe," I say, "but you're meeting him at his best."

She looks around to see if I'm heard. I forget that my voice carries, especially when I try not to be heard, or maybe I don't care who hears.

"You're being uncharitable," she says. But how can she doubt that — she knows who he was and what he's done.

"He doesn't look much different than when I last saw him," I tell her.

"Which was?"

"Well, funny you ask." I turn to her and smile, hardly the sombre look of a son standing by his father's coffin, but something only now has occurred to me. "It was the day we met."

"Who did?"

"You and I."

There's a pause for Nicole to consider whether this is true. I admit to finding her look to be positively endearing as she processes what I've said, replaying, I imagine, the events of that night, only now with the added possibility of things previously unknown to her happening before.

"You're lying," she says, but there's a smile from her, too.

"No. You remember I told you Bruce and I were in Kitchener for a poker game?"

"That was on a Friday. The night before we met."

"Uh-huh. But we spent the night, and the next morning I asked Bruce to swing by my sister's for a quick visit. Mom and Dad had a granny flat there. This was before Dad's Alzheimer's completely took over, but it was far along enough that he couldn't tell which one of us was his son — Bruce or me."

My dad lies there unhearing, and yet it feels like he's taking in every word.

"It was really strange. Mom did all the talking, and Dad just leaned on the kitchen counter wearing the exact same suit he's wearing now, and with a full-on, full-face grin like a happy toddler who hasn't yet learned to talk. 'Course, it didn't help that Bruce and I had a bit of a weed hangover from the night before."

"Of course, this is the first I'm hearing about it."

"Of course. I just remembered."

"How can you forget something like that?"

I tilt my head, shrugging with one shoulder. "To be fair, I didn't know until a few days ago that it would be that last time I'd see him. I almost didn't show up, you know."

"To your father's funeral?"

"No. To our date."

Nicole stares at me for a moment.

"Really?"

"Yeah."

"Asshole. I changed my clothes three times before leaving."

"Oh, that's nice. My dad's funeral and you call me an asshole. Very supportive." But my sarcasm fades away and goes ignored.

"He'll be back," she says of my dad, her eyes lingering on his face longer than I imagined she'd care to see him. "There are too many ghosts in your family." She doesn't believe in ghosts, but she does believe in the panic attacks, the depression, and the insomnia that the dead will sometimes leave in their wake.

I sense someone approaching us. It's Anna's boy, my nephew Jeremy, who puts his hand on my shoulder. "Hi, Uncle Thom," he says, giving Nicole and me a warm condolence hug.

"Ironic, isn't it," I say to Jeremy, "that after all these years your grandfather finally found a way to get us back to church. You think he'd have died sooner if he knew it was going to be this easy." Jeremy laughs, but a look from my sister, his mother, shut him down. *Such responsibility it is to not find humour with the dead.*

The funeral service is about to begin. The pastor fastens the top button of his suit jacket as he moves to take his place at the podium. His deep navy-blue suit is in sharp contrast with the tousle of angel-white hair that tops his head; hair that is slightly unkempt, like that of a man who has fallen asleep in the middle of someone else's sermon. He has the appearance of the everyman, a small-town mayor opening the county fair or a local merchant willing to give you a square deal — an uncomplicated journeyman with a hearty appetite for home-cooked meals and a weakness for freshly baked apple pie.

The pastor looks over the congregation. Beneath him, at the foot of the raised stage, one of his parishioners is lying cold in an open casket, a chalky complexion poised for serenity, arms folded at his chest over his best blue suit. Others have talked about how peaceful he looks, as though he were asleep or deep in meditation. *Dad would think meditation a sin.*

I see a man. Lying in his coffin. As peaceful as a prayer. A man smirking at the crimes he got away with.

Nicole gives, I notice, a cursory glance to see the face of her father-in-law, a man who has affected her life in ways she is still trying to comprehend. It's possible, maybe easier, for her to despise him, because she never had to deal with his intermittent acts of kindness, those joyous moments that kept him afloat, kept him the head of the family, all those things that threw us off just enough to confuse us all. Even I, who feel many things about my father, can't quite find the courage to hate him.

We have a front row pew: my wife, my sisters, their husbands, my mother, and me. We are seated in a place of honour. Behind us sit my nephews, Dennis, David, and Jeremy, and my nieces, Melody and Bethany, with their spouses. Cousins, aunts, uncles are scattered everywhere. Some I recognize, some I've forgotten. There are no children at this funeral. The pastor glances down, assuring eye contact, a trick of the trade, engaging us one at a time before finding my mother, conveniently — or perhaps strategically — the last person seated in our row. This is for her: the things he says, the knowing nods, the comforting smiles. I don't imagine that any of it is for me. I'm probably seen as the proverbial lost son, mired in rock music, drinking, premarital (and sometimes unconventional) sex, smoking, and with a very good chance of having engaged in illicit drug use (they'd be right), but this may be a fabrication of my own guilt. My sisters, from what I know, stay innocent save for one's conversion to Catholicism and the other's hedonistic trips to Las Vegas and to all-inclusive tropical resorts.

In this crowd, I'm the sinner. I don't imagine that the pastor is unaware of my neglect of an aged and sickly man, breaking the commandment that demands me to honour my father. The responsibility of caring for my parents falls to my sisters and their husbands. I, being the youngest and the most irresponsible, am not burdened with that sense of duty. And I certainly felt no obligation to maintain any contact with my father. It didn't have to be like this, but this is what it became.

"Today he is in paradise," the pastor says to my mother, as if the words are only between him and her. *A private joke for members only.* But we hear them, too, my sisters and I and the rest of the congregation, and I suspect only I doubt the words as gospel truth, not just as a matter conflicting with science but of conflicting with the very theology of which he preaches. The pastor's smile broadens, and he shakes his head once in a manner that expresses the unlimited, amazing, and bountiful glory of the Lord. *That precious gift of death.*

"Hallelujah," he says re-enacting an overwhelming fascination with the miracle of death by clutching tight to the side of the podium, tilting his head upward with eyes clenched. "Hallelujah," he says again, this time with a nod. "Hallelujah. Today we bond together in love, in sadness, and in joy." He pauses. Charisma paces itself with anticipation from words chosen and silence selected.

"Oh, what sadness but, oh, what joy. Joy knowing that today Clare is at the side of his maker. Standing in the glory of God's light. Today our brother Clare takes his rightful place in heaven, receiving the Lord's eternal grace. The promise fulfilled by the scripture that says, 'Whosoever believeth in him should not perish, but have eternal life.'"

The grand gestures, the overt praise, the ecstatic shivers — I'm forced to suppress a laugh.

Nicole nudges me. I can't imagine the eternal bliss part. I can only imagine the empty dead part. Were he to have died when I was a child, perhaps I would have had the fantasy of him looking down at me from the heavens. Now I only think of him as gone. I sense the cold of the dead, the vacant shell of a body no longer with the mechanics of life pumping through its veins. The stone I thought of as his heart stopped rattling inside his chest. Dead. Forever. But life eternal?

It's hard to find meaning in my father's death. I look for something significant: an emotion, a change, a sense of relief, a sense of regret, but there's nothing. My father's death makes no more sense to me than his life. He's been gone long enough, anyway, for this final absence to barely register as new. Alzheimer's took him years ago.

And what changes will his death bring? A sudden void in our lives? Not in mine. I can't speak for others.

* * *

Nicole and I talk about this in the car after the service, on our way to my sister's with, as usual, Nicole driving and me in the passenger seat staring out the side window. I fell out of the habit of driving in recent years, for no reason other than Nicole uses the car more than I, and it was just a natural progression for her to take over driving duties, ditching yet another traditional male/female role. I'm okay with this, although, as we anticipated, it hasn't gone unnoticed by my family. It's the kind of role reversal that sets me apart from the rest of the clan and prompts whispered gossip that trails along a line of cousins and aunts and uncles.

Nicole keeps a soft focus on the road ahead. The sun reflecting off the snow-covered fields illuminates the sky with summer warmth and a glare that blends the edges that define landscape from sky.

"Can you get my sunglasses out of my purse?" she asks, removing the glasses she has on and handing them to me. She has a blue canvas shoulder bag the size of a portable DVD carrier that she keeps behind the driver's seat. I find the glasses case that looks like a Gucci rip-off, unzip it, and pull out her sunglasses, replacing them with the ones she handed me. In her sunglasses, she looks to me like a European movie star, and I tell her so, but she's immune to flattery. She is, without question, too beautiful for me.

It may not be the most prominent thought in my mind, but I do recognize that today is as significant to Nicole as it is to me, this death of a man she has only laid eyes on only moments before, lying in his coffin. We take the back roads to my sister's home, where I had spent the night before, and where we would be spending one more night before heading back to Toronto.

The back roads are clear of snow, salted, and ice-free. Winter works better in the country than it does in the city. The empty fields around the roads, the occasional row of pine and spruce trees, everything in a pure white, without the soot of daily traffic and slushy imprints from a parade of muddied boots and galoshes, every now and then a farmhouse and barn set back from the road in a picturesque pose, with cylinder silos standing alongside like castle turrets. I can't see a silo without thinking how as a child I used to think, to the great delight of my parents, that they were rocket ships.

Thom Ernst

And then I tell Nicole about the night before, how I had been in Val and Wayne's dining room working on a short story — a kind of *It's a Wonderful Life* rip-off, except that the protagonist in my story was not guided through his past by an angel but driven by a desire for revenge and justice. Not quite Frank Capra's Christmas classic. Valerie and Wayne were in the living room watching television. The news was on. Valerie called me in to join them. I wasn't getting much done on the story, anyway, so I did. A newscast about Michael Jackson came on. The newscaster commented on a few of Jackson's recent child abuse allegations, followed by Jackson countering the accusations with Peter Pan–like innocence and naïveté.

"I don't know what I'd do if anything like that happened to my boys. Would you?" my sister asked.

I didn't know how to answer. Not right away. This question from Valerie, the only person in the family I'd ever confided in? "I'd be angry," I answer, meeting her eye, hoping to find unspoken understanding reflected to me.

She nods. "I would make sure whoever it was went to jail."

Now, as I tell this story to Nicole, to get the moment out of my head, I'm not expecting Nicole to respond.

I certainly don't expect her to understand. But she's careful. She's thoughtful.

"Are you sure you told her?" she asks.

"Yes. Of course, I told her."

There's a long enough silence to make me think that perhaps the subject has been forgotten. The snow-white fields continue to pass by the window, their very stillness confirming that there is nothing left to say.

"But when was that? You were nineteen." Nicole finally speaks, keeping her eyes on the road.

I look over at her briefly; a bit surprised that she remembers the story that clearly. There's softness in her face that I'm finding quite

220

lovely — the same gentleness I see in her when I think of the days just after we met. I can still be suddenly surprised by how beautiful she is.

"Yes. So?"

"Maybe she forgot. Or maybe she thought you were nineteen and rebellious. Maybe she didn't believe you. Maybe you have to tell her again."

She's right. It makes sense. I assume everyone knows, when perhaps no one does. Or no one remembers. Or no one believes. I look away from Nicole and back into the bright snow blanketing the fields around us.

"That was the absolute perfect thing to say," I tell her, and I think, maybe this is a compliment she takes to heart.

* * *

"Was it all that bad?" Mother asks.

The tough question right out of the gate.

Mom allows me time to hang up my coat, an overpriced Irish-tweed pea jacket that rarely enjoys the luxury of a hanger, let alone a closet. We're at Valerie's now — her home so immaculately organized and tidy that a coat draped over a chair would be as unseemly as a pair of discarded underpants. I turn to take Nicole's coat, a bit of a fraudulent performance since I'm fully aware of Nicole's disdain for most acts of chivalry, although I believe she quietly still expects it. It's a bit of old-school play-acting I've seen my dad do many times with my mother, but only on days when he was wearing a suit and Mom was decked out in one of her finer dresses and wearing the only piece of jewellery I've ever known her to wear: a string of fake pearls.

I'm stalling, of course. *Was it all that bad? Is that what she asked?*

Nicole grants me the opportunity to play the gentleman. She stands with coat in hand, her gloves, hat, and scarf tucked into the sleeve. Hers is a green wool coat as thick and patterned as a carpet-bag. I convinced her to buy it from an upscale boutique we came across while in some city in Normandy when visiting a friend's art installation. It was not an extravagant purchase, but the situation around buying it always makes it seem as if it were extravagant.

Was it all that bad? she had asked.

It shouldn't take this long to hang up a coat, but I need the time to think of a response. I push aside a row of winter outerwear, creating a rush of metal brushing along metal, finding my own coat and hanging Nicole's alongside mine. *Together forever — in summer, winter, and spring.*

Was it all that bad?

So, was it all that bad? Well, yes it was, but is that the real question?

What she's asking is, now that you've outlived him, can we safely say you won and let bygones be bygones? What she's asking is: Is he forgiven?

There's an assumption that with death — his death — all grievances die, too, and the survivor — me — is expected to lay down the gauntlet and acknowledge the dead as though he were an honoured rival. The graveside equivalent of opposing sports teams shaking hands at the end of a match. But I'm not much of a sportsman, and besides, the other team didn't play fair. Shaking hands is out of the question.

I hadn't seen my mother in months before the funeral. She's different in ways I'm unable to pinpoint. Bigger. Older. Slower. Sadder. Wearing the shock of grief and sudden loss. But there's more. She's caught in a moment between the rise and the fall — the millisecond that hangs in mid-air. Held in a place that's neither up nor down. I think of an actor standing in the wings waiting for a cue to be called onstage, no longer herself but not yet in character.

It's been days since Dad died. There has been no burial. Not yet. Dead in the dead of a Canadian winter. Burial put on hold, leaving his body somewhere to lie (appropriately contained and concealed) until the spring thaws the cold, cold ground and once again the earth can receive its own.

Nicole moves with the momentum of someone desperate to forge ahead and avoid the gridlock. She steps between Mom and me, breaking our gaze and buying me a few moments to consider an answer.

"How are you, Margaret?" Nicole asks, touching my mother's shoulder.

"Oh, you know," Mom answers, not wholly committed to playing the martyr but living the moment all the same.

"It's hard. I know," Nicole offers before moving into the kitchen where Wayne is pouring us both a glass of white. She looks at me, her fingertips sliding off my mother's shoulder, her eyes inviting me to take her lead. A mildly seductive glance daring me to let the question go unanswered. But I hesitate too long. I watch her disappear into the next room. I see Valerie already in an apron, pulling together platters of fruits and snacks. My mother's eyes are still fixed on mine. Does her question want an answer? I know what's expected of me. I'm to be kind, console a grieving widow. It is she who lost a husband, not me who lost a father.

Was it all bad? All of it? There was this: rides in the belly of the wheelbarrow, holding on its metal edges as he races over the tiny moguls in the lawn that run from the garden to the garage; the pushes on the swing that get so high I fear I might be flung up and over the bars; the helicopter rides where I'm the propeller held by my arms or legs, sometimes an arm and a leg, and spun until I'm airborne, then he lands me safely back to earth always careful not to hurt me. There are the piggyback rides that I call horsey-back rides, because no one rides on the back of a pig, where I get jostled and bounced down the hall and up again, and there are rides on his shoulders where the real thrill is in being taller than I could ever possibly be. There are the games of crazy eights we would play when he was on morning shifts and was already home when I arrived back from school. There are trips to the drive-in to see Carry On gang movies, Mom and Dad's favourite, where the same cast repeat their roles in every movie no matter if the setting is in a modern department store, a hospital, the army, a ship, the jungle, or ancient Egypt. And even Mom laughs at the scenes where buxom blonds get caught naked and frantically try to cover up; so silly, so British. Dad also takes me to see the Clint Eastwood Man with No Name movie marathon. By this time Mom has stopped going to the drive-in with us. I love them all from *A Fistful of Dollars* to *For a Few Dollars More* to *The Good, the Bad and the Ugly*. He thinks they're too violent. He doesn't like violence; not in the movies, anyway. There's enough violence in the world, he says. He knows because he was alive during the Second World War.

There were things that made him stand out from everyone else; things that made him unique, comical, and quite a character. There were things he did that would draw you near. He spent an inordinate amount of time making sure his two acres of land looked as pristine as a golf course and would shovel the snow off the driveway until there was nothing to see but asphalt. He was immune to the ridicule from those who wouldn't dream of standing outside their homes playing something as unrefined and noisy as the bagpipes, and with such passion and pride uninhibited by the attention the high-pitched notes drew from the neighbours. Clancy would wail and howl, the two acres of open space no buffer for the havoc the bagpipes were playing on her ears. Her agony, her yelping protest accompanying every note was as much part of the performance as the sound of the pipes itself.

There were music nights in the backyard lit by the glow of an inside light from the breezeway. The lawn chairs arranged in a circle so we could sit like cowboys warming at a fire. Uncle Bob played the guitar and sang sad songs about little boys and their lost dogs. "Old Shep" is the song I loved best. My uncle's perfectly pitched baritone voice gave the tune an extra push of melancholy, and Dad strummed along on his Hawaiian guitar, an electric contraption that sat on his lap like a wired keyboard, strung with thick strings too taut and heavy to pluck without a pick, and a metal bar that slid up and down the neck so each note reverberated with an Aloha twang. Later, Valerie would liven things up with the accordion.

These were the times when Dad was part of the team that made sure I was properly fed, clothed, and got enough sleep. Parents who taught me the right way to behave, to be kind, and to mind my manners. They made sure I had regular visits to the dentist, they drove me to the doctor's, they looked after me when I was sick. Parenting. Not allowing me to have too much candy, making sure I dressed warmly when it was cold, wore a hat when it was sunny, slathered on suntan lotion so I didn't get burned, and mosquito repellent so I didn't get eaten alive, went to school (although education was a low priority over a quick and steady paycheque), ate a balanced meal, had a good breakfast, and learned to treat others the way I want to be treated. They took me to church, took me on picnics, took me for walks in the fields behind Montag's farm. They told me about equality, that all men are equal in the eyes of the Lord (except Catholics and Jews and hippies and atheists), and that a gentleman always had a tissue ready when taking a girl to the movies in case the film was sad and she needed something to wipe her tears. They warned me about drugs and alcohol, about shady characters who might lead me astray. They told me the story of a neighbourhood kid named Jimmy who jumped out of a moving car after accepting a ride from a stranger who meant to do him harm. Jimmy knew he was in danger because he saw the man reaching for the knife he had hidden in the car seat. Jimmy was lucky he got away with just a broken arm. He became a local hero, and I couldn't wait until I was old enough to hitchhike so I could get picked up by stranger who meant me harm and jump out of the car. (But the person who meant me harm wasn't a stranger.) They taught me not to slouch, to be kind to children, to obey the law and respect the police (but don't become one because no one likes police officers). I knew not to steal, not to run into traffic, not to swim too far from the shore, not to ride my bike at night without a light. They prepared me for the real world, to open a bank account, to think about what I wanted to do when I grow up. To get a good trade like a plumber (because someone always needs a plumber, and by George, those guys get paid a lot), or electrician or carpenter, a steady factory job or, who knows, a salesman in a fancy department store just like my Uncle Quinnie. They hoped I would marry and raise a family of my own.

They did all the things that parents did, out of instinct and love. All the things that parents did to keep their children safe, to help them grow to be strong, healthy, happy, and hopeful. All the things that parents did so that their children found the skills to live in a world that could sometimes seem too hard to live in.

"No," I say to my mother. "It wasn't all bad."

She nods and looks at her hands, as though contemplating a second and even tougher question, but when her eyes lift, she is no longer looking at me but to the side, lost in a thought she isn't able to share.

I believe she is grateful for the lie.

And I'm grateful that she recognizes it as a lie.

Chapter 26

My mother saw another ghost, and it had left her crying through the night.

I hadn't talked to my mother in days. I believe she knew. I believe, too, that she had effectively convinced herself to not know. She had developed ways to survive just as I had, although one of the ways she survived was to leave me alone to face the lion.

My mother is in her nineties now. Lonely, memory slipping, in some ways perhaps conveniently.

Mom admitted to being depressed. This complaint became more frequent.

"Oh, I'm feeling a bit down" had become "I'm just so doggone depressed." She even said that sometimes she wished she were dead.

"It must be hard, but surely you have some friends there," I said, meaning others at the seniors home where she lived. She would spend her days knitting and missing her cat, a white Himalayan named Truman.

We talked about my sisters, and about my sister Anna's husband's cancer, thankfully now in remission. We talked about how everyone in her building was either too old or suffered from dementia. Her only friend, Norma, had been taken to a facility where she could be better cared for. My mother was indeed lonely.

I apologized to her for not calling sooner, but my mother played the martyr and let me off the hook: "Well, you're busy, too."

I don't know whom she meant when she said "too." Her? My sisters? The grandchildren?

But I'm not that busy; I just don't know how to deal with a ninety-five-year-old woman whom I believe turned her back on me when I needed her most. Forgiveness is healing, I am told. But it was forgiveness, or least a close relative to forgiveness, that kept me from telling anyone, that allowed me to wait so long to speak out, that held me back from demanding justice.

My mother told me that late at night someone knocked on her door. The door was unlocked so she told them to come in. "Guess who it was?" she asked. But I didn't have to guess. But neither did I want to hear myself say the words.

"Who?" I asked.

"Dad," she said. "He just walked right in dressed in his suit."

I knew the suit she meant. The blue three-piece suit with the vest and three-button jacket with the lapels jutting out like the tips of ballpoint pens. A handkerchief folded and placed into the left breast pocket. Slight pinstripes running up and down the jacket and the sharply pressed pants. His white shirt with a collar too large to be in fashion, and a two-toned blue tie tied with a Windsor knot.

I saw him in my mind's eye walking into my mother's room as real as an angel outside her bedroom window, as real as a rocking chair moving on its own.

"I cried and cried," Mom said. "I guess I just miss him so much."

Chapter 27

-- -- -- -- -- -- --

Nicole and I have our own little girl now. My own child. What Michelle will make of all this, I can't yet say.

Perhaps there's nothing to make of it at all. Not yet. She's the innocent. She only knows that something in the long past wasn't right; the rest we protect her from. One day she'll have read this book and she'll know; it's all here, at least what I remember of it. And she'll discover for herself and come to her own opinion as to how it happened, why it happened, and what it means. She might cry or be angry. She might blame me, or she might not feel the need to blame anyone at all.

I look at her now, asleep. The glow from a ceramic night light — the one she's had since infancy, depicting a Celtic folklore fairy hovering above an open flower — casts a soft glaze of light across her face, illuminating a faint smile that is either prompted by a contented dream or is the reflex of a child playing a trick on her father. Is she asleep, or just pretending? What if she should open her eyes and see me standing here? Would she stretch and yawn and pull herself into a waking world, or she would scowl and grumble, turn away, hug ladybug even tighter, demanding more sleep?

Either way, my little girl will not be startled, or afraid, or concerned. I'm her father. She trusts me. And that's what breaks my heart: that in one horrifying moment I could break that trust. I have that power. So, when I say she's safe, who am I reassuring? Her or me?

I didn't intend to be here, standing in Michelle's room, bending over her, whispering in her ear, as I am, saying something so innocuous that if someone were to hear, it would seem to make no sense at all.

I had one goal this morning: to get up at the unrighteous hour of 4:30 a.m. on a Sunday morning and make it to my office at the end of a long hall without waking the rest of the family. And without spilling my coffee along the way. I walk down the hallway doing my best comic book prowl, a pantomime of a cat burglar on tiptoes taking slow, deliberate steps. I hold my breath when I get outside the bedrooms, willing myself to be weightless, hoping that gravity is fooled into thinking I'm nowhere near. But gravity is one law that can't be broken nor easily tricked. I know because as kids, Doug, whom I now only see on the rarest of occasions, and I would leap from tree branches and swing sets in the homemade capes his brother Rick made for us, determined to learn how to fly so we could grow up to be superheroes.

I easily pass the room I share with Nicole. Our bedroom door is shut. It's Michelle who keeps her door wide open, leaving no buffer between her sleep and the sound of the floorboards that creak beneath my feet. Floorboards that break the morning silence, resonating with a squawk like rusty hinges pried from wet wood. I stop, poised like a dangling marionette with my arms raised by my sides, holding my coffee cup steady, to give silence a chance to settle back in.

My sleeping child doesn't move. There's not even the false threat that happens in movies where the sleeper snorts and puffs and shifts positions before settling back into their pillow. I should continue down the hall, but now I'm distracted by an unformed memory of something that happened as recent as yesterday. Nothing specific. Just something about my little girl and the things she's able to give me. Her unwavering trust. Her vulnerability. Her unconditional love. All the intangible things that get lost in the moment but that I ache for when she's not around. I stand by Michelle's door, calculating the risk of going into her room without waking her, for no reason but to see her and to appreciate the moment.

There is a second night light that I've forgotten about, a blue five-pointed star pierced with factory-aligned holes and clamped overtop a twenty-watt light bulb mounted on the wall. I worry about fire and check regularly to make sure the star hasn't heated up into a melting blob. It's by this light I get an even better look at the room, allowing me to navigate past any discarded story books or wayward toys that might clutter the pathway between her door and her bed.

It's still not enough light to see her. She's just out of view beneath the canopy of the fortress she's constructed from the frame of a bunk bed — a prefabricated bit of Swedish furniture that lifts her off the ground, leaving extra floor space for dolls and board games and Lego sets.

A few more hours before she wakes. And when she does her eyes will open as if snapped out of hypnosis. Asleep then awake. Nothing in between. No stretching, no yawning, no coming to terms with the real world again. She'll come clumping down the stairs, dragging ladybug behind her, looking for me so we can watch a movie. And she will find me, and we'll cuddle up together on the basement couch watching movies. Maybe it won't be *Tinkerbell* or *My Little Pony*, maybe it'll be a movie based on a collection of her Monster High dolls or something with a talking dog voiced by Chevy Chase, or Jim Belushi, or George Lopez. I'll grumble about her choices, hoping for something ironic like *Uncle Grandpa* or

Adventure Time, but I'll end up watching whatever she chooses. And I usually like them, especially the talking-dog ones — there's inherent cleverness exclusive to the talking-dog genre.

I know I should move on. It's safe to take another step. Many steps and with longer strides. Moving down the hall like a stone skipping across the water, never touching down long enough to sink. But instead, I go into her room. The floor doesn't creak so loudly now, or at least it doesn't seem to.

I move to the head of her bed — a raised loft that meets me at chest level. I smile because it's impossible not to. She sleeps facing north. Always does, as if this too might be a comforting nighttime ritual. Her hair has been brushed from the side of her face and tucked behind her ear. Her eyes are closed. It's a strange feeling to be so close and yet remain invisible.

I lean in to kiss her cheek, maybe her forehead just above the temple, in what would be a selfish act of affection. But then I lean into her ear. I whisper something while she sleeps although her eyelids are pressed so softly together that I wonder if she's clever enough to feign sleep so she can hear what's said by people who believe she's not listening. I expect to say something like "I love you" — hoping my words creep into her dreams. But those aren't the words that come out of me.

I have no idea what I'm about to say until I say it. Until I hear it myself.

"You're safe," I tell her.

This time she stirs, but just a bit, and I want to believe that that's a smile crossing her face. I want to believe that even in her dreams she knows the sound of my voice, and my voice, as simple, as ineffective as my voice can sometimes be, fills her with comfort and trust.

Acknowledgements

A book like *The Wild Boy of Waubamik* is not written without full knowledge that the journey is not done alone. I am indebted to the people whose charity, goodwill, and encouragement brought *The Wild Boy of Waubamik* to the page.

First, to my wife, Nicole, and our daughter, Michelle, who are as much my inspiration as they are my support.

Thank you, too, to Transatlantic and Rob Firing, my agent and friend, for taking me on as a client and for steering me in the right direction at every crossroad.

To my friend and colleague, Johanna Schneller, for reading *Wild Boy* when it was little more than ideas scratched on paper. Johanna's encouragement gave me precisely what I needed to move forward.

To Heidi von Palleske, who went beyond the call of friendship by reading nearly every version of *Wild Boy*, demanding that I take the Queen streetcar to the Dundurn office and hand my manuscript directly to Russell Smith.

Russell Smith, my acquiring editor from Dundurn Press, for seeing the potential in *Wild Boy* and helping me see it.

Thank you to everyone at Dundurn Press: managing editor Elena Radic, who tackled my every unreasonable request, every newbie question, and acted like it was all routine; copy editor Laurie Miller; and proofreader Rachel Spence.

Thank you, Alyssa Boyden, Sara D'Agostino, Laura Boyle, and the entire marketing and publicity team.

A big thank-you to the incredible Jane Warren, who has been making writers look good for decades. Thank you for your talent and your insight.

I wish to thank family members, from both sides of the adoption coin, who shared their memories and stories with me. A special thank-you to my sisters for allowing me to share our story as best as I could.

I thank the many friends and colleagues who have read earlier manuscripts: Heidi von Palleske, Valerie Freund, Matt Gallagher, Cornelia Principe, Jean Dipak Sen, Carol Anderson, Doug Collins, Dennis Freund, Lorrayne Anthony, Any Francois, Jason Wodlinger, Mark Breslin, Jenny Marino, Andrew Pyper, Ian Brown, Pam Syvier, Patty Becker, Chuck Marino, Domenico Capilongo, Richard Crouse, and Dave Bidini.

Thank you to the many friends and organizations who helped fund the project in its early stages of research: the Ontario Arts Council, Sara Marino, Sajid Qureshi, Liz Braun, Viviana Kohon, Dan Riskin, Carol Anderson, Ian Bragg, Angela Tsmentzis, Aaron Leckie, Anson and Genna Bowlby, Zoe Redlich, Elizabeth Payne, Wendy Tutt, Mark Slone, Paul Chetcuti, Patrice Coacolo, Lauretta Stewart, Nikku Nepal, Marty Logan, David Freund, Lisa Blundon, Mikey Murren, Deb B., Josh Morden, David Newland, Nisha Pahuja, Deanna Wilk, James and Renee Laforet, and Austen Valentine.

And for their work in understanding and dealing with the trauma of childhood sexual violence, thank you to Dr. Alan Berwick and Dr. Jane Thurley.

Heartfelt thanks to Arthur, Maria, and everyone at The Gatehouse for your work to help end child sexual violence.

About the Author

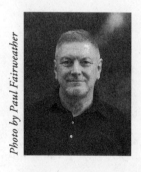

Photo by Paul Fairweather

THOM ERNST is a Toronto based film critic and writer and an active member of the Toronto Film Critics Association. His written work on film has appeared in various publications. Thom is perhaps best remembered as the host, interviewer, and producer of television's longest running movie program, *Saturday Night at the Movies*, and Bell Media's *Making Movies the Canadian Way*. Currently, Thom's film reviews can be read on Original-Cin and Northernstars. He can be heard interviewing Canadian filmmakers on the Kingston Canadian Film Festival podcast, *Rewind Fast Forward*. *The Wild Boy of Waubamik* is Thom's first book.